STROKE
naturally
PREVENTION

PROVEN NON-PHARMACEUTICAL
STROKE AVOIDANCE STRATEGIES

FELIX VELOSO, M.D., F.R.C.P.(C), F.A.A.N.
with Roxanne Veloso-Tang, B.S.P., R.Ph.
illustrated by Natasha Kaitlin Veloso Tang

Stroke Prevention Naturally:
Proven Non-Pharmaceutical Stroke Avoidance Strategies
© Dr. Felix Veloso, M.D., F.R.C.P.(C), F.A.A.N., 2010

Library and Archives Canada Cataloguing in Publication

Veloso, Felix, 1936-
Stroke prevention naturally : proven non-pharmaceutical stroke avoidance strategies /
Felix Veloso ; with Roxanne Veloso-Tang ; illustrated by Natasha Kaitlin Veloso Tang.

Includes bibliographical references and index.
ISBN 978-1-894431-57-6

1. Cerebrovascular disease—Prevention. 2. Lifestyles—Health
aspects. I. Veloso-Tang, Roxanne, 1960- II. Title.

RC388.5.V45 2010   616.8'105   C2010-906551-4

Layout and design by Heather Nickel
Front cover image © Wee Lee
Brain image © ryan burke/www.istockphoto.com

Printed in Canada
November 2010

Your Nickel's Worth Publishing
Regina, SK.

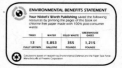

www.yournickelsworth.com

This book is dedicated to my patients
—who taught me the art of medicine—
my wife, Ruby Lim Veloso
my daughters, Roxanne Veloso-Tang and Joanne Veloso
and my granddaughter, Natasha Kaitlin Veloso Tang

table of contents

introduction

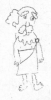

"Nature does nothing uselessly."

~ ARISTOTLE
Greek philosopher (384 BC – 322 BC)

*"I would feel more optimistic about a bright future for man
if he spent less time proving that he can outwit nature and
more time tasting her sweetness and respecting her seniority."*

~ E. B. WHITE
U.S. author (1899 – 1985)

Stroke is the leading cause of permanent disability. It is the second leading cause of death worldwide, with more than 85% of deaths from stroke occurring in developing countries. In Canada, the direct and indirect cost of stroke is at least $3 billion yearly and climbing. The American Heart Association estimated the direct costs of medical care and therapy for stroke in 2004 was $33 billion US and indirect costs from lost productivity was $20.6 billion US, for a total of approximately $54 billion US. In 2001, The National Stroke Association projected the average cost for the first three months per stroke was $15,000

US, although the expense for 10% of the patients was at least $35,000 US.[1]

Latest statistics reveal that pharmaceuticals are the second most expensive component, accounting for 17.4% of the total health cost of 10.7% of the Canadian Gross Domestic Product. Hospitals are the largest component, consuming 28%, and physician fees come in third at 13.4% of total spending. More alarmingly, the cost of pharmaceuticals is inflating the fastest of the three major categories of health care costs—at a rate of 8.3% annually, compared to physicians' pay at 6.2% and hospital spending at 5.8%.

Clinical research comparing a widely prescribed new antiplatelet agent—a medication which helps prevent blood clotting—to aspirin (*acetasalicylic acid* or a.s.a.), showed only an insignificant trend favouring the newer, much more expensive drug over the already proven 2.7% stroke risk reduction established by aspirin. On the basis of the most accurate measurement of cost effectiveness of medical intervention, which is the *number needed to treat* or NNT, researchers determined that for the newer antiplatelet agent the magic number is 115. This means that 115 patients would have to be treated for 730 days (two years) at a cost of $2.75 per tablet in order to prevent one patient from having a stroke. That translates to a cost of $200,750 per stroke prevented. The equivalent cost for aspirin is about $730. A single regular tablet of 325 mg aspirin costs, at most, 10 cents, but one tablet of the heavily promoted newer antiplatelet medication costs approximately $2.75 (28 times more expensive) and is no more effective than aspirin in preventing stroke.[2]

Fortunately, although a growing major public health problem, especially with Canada's increasingly aging population, stroke is not only uniquely preventable but—more importantly—can be simply and naturally avoided without the use of expensive, potentially harmful, pharmaceuticals. A study by Dr. Philip Gorelick titled "Primary Prevention of Stroke: Impact of

Healthy Lifestyle" reported that a prospective cohort study of 43,685 men and 71,243 women found that those with all five low-risk factors:

LOW-RISK FACTORS FOR STROKE

- not smoking
- an ideal body weight
- 30 or more minutes of moderate intensity exercise per day
- modest alcohol consumption of one to two ounces per day
- and eating a healthy diet of vegetables, fruits, low-fat dairy products and lean meats

had a substantial stroke reduction of up to 80% compared with those who had none of the factors. And what is even more impressive is the INTERSTROKE research, a Canadian-led study, suggesting that 90% of the 10 stroke risk factors:

STROKE RISK FACTORS

- high blood pressure
- smoking
- abdominal obesity
- unhealthy diet
- physical inactivity
- high cholesterol
- diabetes mellitus
- alcohol abuse
- stress/depression
- and heart disease[3]

are preventable through lifestyle changes. In other words, a healthy lifestyle can prevent up to 90% of strokes.

Most remarkably, healthy lifestyle prevents both primary and recurrent strokes, and the cost of adopting a healthy lifestyle is free! It is also important to remember that antiplatelet agents provide only secondary or recurrent stroke prevention. The internationally recognized authoritative *Cochrane Reviews*,[4] which investigates the evidence-based cost-effectiveness of medical interventions, concluded that the differences between *clopidogrel* and aspirin, in terms of the outcomes of total strokes and total deaths, are not significant. This is just one example of the high cost of potentially harmful pharmaceuticals that should convince even the most skeptical that nature's way is not only the best but is also freely available to everybody who wants it.

Readers of this book will learn simple and easy-to-adopt strategies on natural, healthy, lifestyle changes that will allow them to prevent stroke and its equally devastating twin disease of heart attack, as well as to avoid dementia—especially of the type related to stroke, commonly known as vascular or multi-infarct dementia.

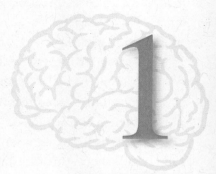

why natural?

"The goal of life is living in agreement with nature."

~ ZENO
Greek philosopher (335 BC – 264 BC)

"The best six doctors anywhere
and no one can deny it
are sunshine, water, rest, and air
exercise and diet.
These six will gladly you attend
if only you are willing
your mind they'll ease
your will they'll mend
and charge you not a shilling."

~ ANONYMOUS

Poisons are substances that harm by interfering with the normal structure or function of our bodies. All drugs are poisons since they interfere with the normal physical or physiological activities that keep us healthy. The risks of drugs are directly

proportional to cost, while the benefits are inversely proportional. A single regular tablet of 325 mg aspirin (*acetasalicylic
acid* or a.s.a.) costs as little as 10 cents. One tablet of a new platelet anti-aggregant costs approximately $2.75, about 28 times
more and is, at best, only marginally more effective than aspirin
in preventing stroke, but with greater risk of serious damage to
your white blood cells. Recent studies also show that, contrary
to expectation, the additional of clopidogrel to aspirin does
not prevent more strokes or heart attacks but rather *increases*
risk of serious bleeding complications. In fact, the "Clopidogrel
for High Athero-thrombotic Risk and Ischemia Stabilization,
Management, and Avoidance (CHARISMA)" study involving
15,603 patients with heart disease or multiple risk factors for
heart disease, published in the prestigious *New England Journal of Medicine*, showed that adding clopidogrel to aspirin doubles heart disease deaths among patients who had not yet had
a heart attack but who had multiple risk factors, such as high
blood pressure and diabetes.[5]

Diuretics, particularly the potassium-sparing type (which do
not promote the secretion of potassium into the urine and are
used in the treatment of hypertension and the management of
congestive heart failure to maintain a normal range for potassium), reduce the risk of developing Alzheimer's disease by up
to 70%, compared to the much more expensive antihypertensive medication, such as angiotensin converting enzyme (ACE)
inhibitors, or the even newer and more expensive angiotensin
receptor blockers, which reduce risk by only 40%, according to
a study involving 3,200 elderly Utah residents funded by the
National Institute of Health.[6]

Be wary of "randomized double–blind controlled studies"
because these types of research are designed to prove that a
drug is effective on carefully selected patients. It may not apply
to the general population and it does not focus on the side effects of the drug.

Nature has been perfecting itself since the beginning of time. The development of pharmaceuticals, as we know them today, started only about a century ago. In earlier times, mankind survived both plagues and pestilence using only the herbs available in nature.

Drugs are made by man. Drugs have side effects. Most times the side effects are mild but rarely they can be deadly. Witness Baycol® (a cholesterol-lowering agent) and Voixx® (an anti-inflammatory), just two of the latest examples.[7]

The process of making drugs starts with the identification of a chemical that is usually similar to another compound already shown to be effective for a particular condition. The agent then undergoes phase one studies to determine the metabolism and pharmacologic actions of the drug in humans, usually normal subjects. The promising agent then goes to phase two, in which studies are conducted to determine the most effective dose with the least number of side effects for the condition being treated. If the compound still shows promise and the side effects are "tolerable or not serious" (for which read "did not kill or disable") then the drug enters phase three study, the pivotal expanded trial to gather additional information regarding the overall benefit-risk relationship of the drug in preparation for filing with regulatory authorities for approval to market it. Notice that the whole process—from the initial identification of the compound to the final approval for marketing—needs only evidence showing that the drug is effective, even marginally, without "known serious side effect." Is it any wonder then that patients are demanding to treat their health problems "natur*ally*"?

The advent of the Internet, and the invention of near-magical imaging procedures such as *computerized axial tomography (CAT)* and *magnetic resonance imaging (MRI)* scans, and the availability of numerous versions of the same class of dubiously effectivene medication for a variety of diseases have provided such a bewildering wealth of information that health care professionals sometimes (and patients often!) have problems understanding the best treatment option. Take, for example, the numerous types and brands of the same kind of antibiotics in your local pharmacy. Additionally, patients are now much more educated and sophisticated, and rightfully demand to participate in the decision-making process regarding their health care. This practice inevitably leads to self-diagnosis and treatment, a frightening prospect for anyone, particularly a sick person in search of help. It should therefore be obligatory for the caring physician to consult with a fully informed patient to ensure that a mutually agreed treatment plan is implemented.

In my more than 40 years of practice as a clinical neurologist, I have been impressed by the great number of patients who intuitively felt a tremendous aversion to drugs ("pills or chemicals") and prefer natural or non-prescription medications for treatment of their illnesses. This is especially true of stroke victims and their loved ones, who understandably long for "anything that could have been done" natur*ally* to prevent the stroke.

Studies continue to confirm that a healthy lifestyle reduces the risk of stroke by up to 90%. There is no drug currently available that can provide similar benefit, regardless of the cost of the medication. These natural remedies also avert heart attack since these two conditions share similar pathophysiology and often coexist—up to 40% of stroke patients already have significant silent heart disease and from 2-5% have a heart attack within 90 days of their stroke. Moreover, evidence is rapidly accumulating that these natural, non-pharmaceutical strategies reduce dementia, particularly of the mixed type—a combination of Alzheimer's disease and vascular dementia. This is because neuroscientists continue to discover that stroke and dementia share similar risk factors so that prevention of one also avoids the other. It is now increasingly evident that a healthy lifestyle naturally protects the structural integrity of our wondrous brain that weighs only three pounds (1.6% of the average north American male weight of 190 pounds) but also ensures that its 1,000 billion neurons and its 1,000 trillion connections function normally so that we maintain our cognitive uniqueness among living creatures.

Natural medicine necessarily uses herbs, spices and other plant nutrients to prevent and treat ailments. It is therefore important that we have a basic understanding of *pharmaconogsy*, the study of medicines derived from natural sources.

Most medicinal herbs contain many natural compounds that play off one another, producing a wide variety of results. Even medical science does not always understand how the compounds work together, or even exactly what they all are. As botanist Walter Lewis, Ph.D., and microbiologist Memory Elvin-Lewis, Ph.D., put it in their book *Medical Botany*: "Nature is still mankind's greatest chemist, and many compounds that remain undiscovered in plants are beyond the imagination of even our best scientists."[8]

Some herbs that regulate the body seem to almost have an inner intelligence, with the ability to perform many different functions depending upon what the individual needs. For example, **ginger** can raise or lower blood pressure, depending on what needs to happen to bring an individual's blood pressure to a healthy level. And tonic herbs do more than clear up immediate, acute symptoms—they have the more general effect of renewing strength and vitality. **Marshmallow**, for instance, strengthens your digestive system and improves the functioning of your immune system while relieving your stomach distress.

Although 80% of pharmaceutical drugs are based on herbs, these drugs are generally based not on the *whole* herb but on one "active ingredient" derived from a plant. Modern medicine has become captivated by what it calls a "magic bullet"—a single substance that zeros in and destroys a germ or relieves a symptom. Whenever possible, the chemical structure of the active component found in an herb is duplicated in the laboratory and produced synthetically. This enables a drug company to produce formulas of consistent quality and strength, and avoid the hassle and expense of collecting plants in the wild. Not incidentally, it also enables them to patent the remedy and charge more money for it.

These magic bullet drugs have several issues. First, they treat only specific problems. Well-known plant researcher and botanist James Duke, Ph.D., points out that "the solitary synthetic bullet offers no alternatives if the doctor has misdiagnosed the ailment or if one or more ailments require more than one compound."[9] And Francois Voltaire's cynically, if not candidly, observed that "Physicians pour drugs of which they know little, to cure diseases of which they know less, into humans of which they know nothing." Herbs, on the other hand, can cover many bases at once.

Magic bullets don't give the body a chance to find its own solution. Dr. Duke theorizes that our bodies take fuller advantage than we realize of the complex chemistry in medicinal herbs. He believes that each herb contains hundreds of active compounds, many of which act "synergistically." That means that all these compounds somehow combine to produce a greater effect than each has alone, and that the body extracts the compounds it needs and discards the others. One possible reason that scientific studies sometimes fail to confirm an herb's traditional use in healing is that the studies often focus only on the isolated compound, not on the whole plant.

Years ago, researchers extracted an active compound called *silymarin* from the herb **milk thistle** and turned it into a pharmaceutical drug to treat liver damage. Only later did German scientists discover yet another compound in milk thistle—*betaine hydrochloride*—that may be equally important.

The popular immunity-enhancing herb **echinacea** has a similar story. For years, complex carbohydrates from echinacea were thought to be its sole active ingredients and were extract-ed to produce a drug. But then a team of German researchers headed by Dr. Wagner discovered that echinacea contains other compounds that also enhance immunity.

In the case of the sedative herb **valerian**, medical research-ers found that two compounds—*valeric acid* and *essential oils*—caused its calming effects, but for some time they remained un-aware of still a third set of highly sedative compounds called *valepotriates*. And **ginkgo**, which is used to boost brain func-tions and circulation, has been found to be more effective when used in its whole form instead of its isolated active compounds. In an ideal medical system, *herbalism* would be viewed as a legitimate medical therapy, not as an outside or "alternative" therapy. Recently, instruction in herbal therapy has been inte-grated into some medical curricula in Germany.

So there is hope.

Unfortunately, in North America, medicine is extremely drug-oriented. It is therefore not surprising that doctors, who are trained to use drugs, are hesitant to study herbs. Herbalist Michael Moore, author of *Medicinal Plants of the Pacific West*, sums it up well: "I have known perfectly intelligent physicians whose sole regularly used reference manuals were the *Physician's Desk Reference* and *Goodman & Gillman*, both drug manuals. Their patients have come to expect, and receive, prescriptions as their only therapy."[10]

Obviously, doctors are not the only ones who consider drugs their first option for treatment. Pharmaceutical companies are just as unlikely to change the way they do business. They can easily spend anywhere from $50 million to $100 million, mostly for safety testing, when submitting a new drug application to the United States Federal Drug Administration for approval. These companies are willing to pay that much because a new drug can reap incredible profits for the firm holding the drug's patent rights. Herbs, however, are available to anyone with a garden, and they cannot be patented. Drug companies are understandably reluctant to invest in a product that competitors can pick up after the research is done. The result is that few herbal remedies are manufactured commercially, and drug use (especially use of specific brands of drugs) is encouraged.

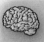 ***Compelling Reasons to Use Natural Remedies***

- General disillusionment with modern medicine
- High cost and side effects of prescription drugs
- Wide availability of low- or no-cost natural remedies
- The belief that "nature-made" remedies are superior to man-made drugs
- Newly-gained knowledge of the benefits of healthy lifestyle living

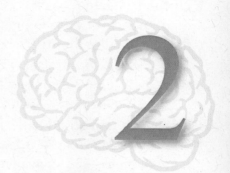

strokes deprive

"Everyone ought to be his own physician."

~ GREEK PROVERB

I was halfway through my customary 16-kilometre Sunday morning jog in Wascana Centre—which, at 2,325 acres, is the ninth largest urban park in the world—when my cell phone rang, sounding like the siren of an ambulance. It was a beautiful sunny spring day in May. The air was perfumed with the fragrance of blooming lilacs and filled with music from a myriad of singing birds that populate the trees around Wascana Lake. The Canada geese and newly hatched goslings were enjoying tender shoots of grass while robins feasted on earthworms dug up in their wake. Fellow ParticipACTIONers were actively deriving health benefits from walking, jogging and biking on the pathway surrounding postcard-perfect Wascana Lake.

"This is the General Hospital Emergency Room. Dr. Emerge needs to talk to you immediately," the nurse said after I confirmed being on-call for neurology. Dr. Phil Emerge is the greatly respected director of the Emergency Department who encouraged and advised our group of neurologists, neurosurgeons, radiologists, cardiologists, physiatrists (physical medicine/rehabilitation specialists), internists and vascular surgeons for almost three years to organize a state-of-the-art stroke unit that had finally admitted its first stroke patient just three weeks earlier. I knew from past experience that when Dr. Emerge said *immediately*, he really meant *emergency*.

"Felix, I have a Mr. Victor Patience here who had a stroke about an hour ago. His wife, Prudence, happened to attend the stroke meeting you presented two weeks ago (*And a good thing too,* I thought—she knew that a stroke is a brain attack and like heart attack is a medical emergency that must be treated immediately to reduce permanent brain damage). She called 9-1-1 about an hour ago when her husband collapsed with left-sided weakness while smoking his third cigarette of the day and drinking his second cup of coffee. He arrived here about 10 minutes ago. He is completely paralyzed on the left side, but is fully awake and responsive to command. His blood pressure is 220/120 and his pulse rate is regular at 88 per minute," Dr. Emerge informed me.

I quickly calculated that we had—at most—110 minutes left to complete the many clinical, laboratory and radiologic evaluations needed to safely administer *tissue plasminogen activator (tPA)* that Health Canada has approved for the treatment of acute stroke. TPA is the only evidence-based treatment for acute stroke. Studies show that tPA provides one out of every 12 treated patients with complete functional recovery from a disabling stroke if administered within three hours of stroke symptom onset. The same studies also show that life saving tPA has a serious side effect of increasing the risks of serious brain hemorrhage by up to 10 times.[11] This potentially deadly bleeding complication of tPA is much, and unacceptably, higher if administered more than three hours after stroke onset. That is why accurate timing of stroke onset is critically important.

There are several other equally important but perhaps less serious issues that must be considered before administering intravenous tPA as well, as you'll see.

"Is Mrs. Patience nearby? I need more information from her immediately," I asked Dr. Emerge.

"Where is Mrs. Patience?" I overheard Dr. Emerge ask the nurse.

"She's in the waiting room."

"Go get her. Dr. Veloso needs to talk to her right now," Dr. Emerge told the nurse.

After an agonizing minute or so, Mrs. Patience came on the line. "Is that you, Dr. Veloso? Do you remember me? I was the one who asked about snake venom as a stroke treatment at your presentation two weeks ago."

How could I forget the sixty-ish grey-haired lady who had asked a question that astounded me with her knowledge of the latest in stroke research, but which elicited laughters from audience members, who'd apparently thought she was being funny.

"Yes, Mrs. Patience, I definitely remember you. I will be over there right away," I replied. "But first I must know if your husband has had a head injury or major surgery recently, as either one of these conditions automatically disqualifies him from receiving tPA."

"No, Dr. Veloso. Victor has not had any head trauma or operations for at least a few years," Mrs. Patience guaranteed.

That was good news. "Please let me talk to Dr. Emerge again," I requested. He came back on the line. "Phil, I am on my way. Please give Mr. and Mrs. Patience the Informed Consent Form for tPA treatment to read and sign as soon as possible. Also, notify the stroke nurse, Florence Strokeller, of Mr. Patience's arrival and status so she can help assess him for tPA treatment," I told the emergency room physician.

Shortly after the board of directors approved the stroke unit; the Regional Health Authority had appointed a stroke nurse to coordinate the activities of the in-patient, eight-bed stroke unit and a weekly, outpatient stroke clinic.

When on-call, I jogged only along the perimeter of the Wascana Centre, about one kilometre from the City General Hospital. My white, front-wheel drive Rabbit was parked approximately half a mile away. A quick calculation determined that I would waste precious minutes by running to my car first and driving to the hospital, so I raced to the hospital on foot, reaching the emergency room in only minutes. It was not the record-breaking, first-ever, less-than-four-minute-mile run of my idol and fellow neurologist, Dr. Roger Bannister, which had taken place almost 50 years earlier, but it was and remains my personal best of six minutes-to-the-mile. On the way, I reviewed the circumstances in which I'd met Mrs. Patience and the discussion I'd had two weeks earlier with an audience of mostly retirees in a question-and-answer session titled, "Time is Brain."

"I'm sure you will be pleased to know that the long-awaited state-of-the-art stroke unit, dedicated to the treatment of the first cause of permanent disability, is now open to admit stroke patients," I had told the Provincial Visible Minority Employees Association annual meeting where I had been invited to discuss the most serious health problem facing our rapidly aging population. I had informed the audience that the Stroke Prevention and Management Unit had been three years in the planning. There were other stroke units, but all were in academic centres and most had been created for research purposes. The new Regional Health Authority stroke unit was the only one dedicated to patient care.

"Stroke is a growing major but increasingly preventable disease," I had said. "The occurrence of stroke is growing because of our rapidly aging population and age is its most significant risk factor. It has been estimated that the incidence of stroke more than doubles in each successive decade of life over age 55. Think of the baby boomers rapidly reaching retirement age and you can easily see the exploding prevalence of stroke in the near future. Seventy-two per cent of victims of stroke are older than 65. Twenty-five per cent—one in four Canadians—will be 65 or older by 2056, which is two times the current rate of 13% or one in eight.

"The good news is that stroke is arguably the easiest of the three foremost killing diseases to prevent. Although stroke is the third largest cause of death in Canada (heart attack is first and cancer, second) and second around the world, it is the second highest cause of dementia and, most distressing, is the leading cause of disability in the western world. Nearly one in every 14 deaths is attributable to stroke and 75,000 new strokes occur annually. Approximately 16,000 people died from acute stroke in 1998; almost half of these deaths occurred out of hospital.

"Of those who survive an initial stroke, 25% will die within a year. The average post-stroke survival rate for stroke victims is seven years. There were 4.4 million stroke survivors in the U.S. in 1998. Recovery from a stroke depends on its severity. Fifteen per cent to 30% of survivors remain permanently disabled. Fourteen per cent of those who have a first stroke or a *transient ischemic attack (TIA)* will have another stroke within one year. There are approximately 450,000 stroke survivors alive in Canada today. More than 200,000 of them live with the crippling and lifelong disabilities of paralysis, loss of speech and poor memory.[12] Health care professionals predict that simply reducing the risks of stroke can prevent 90% of all strokes within 10 years. In this meeting, you will learn safe, free, practical, adaptable, easy strategies that health scientists have identified to prevent stroke naturally."[13]

"Can you please put that in perspective?" asked one of the 500 or so people attending the seminar that beautiful spring day.

"I'll try," I answered. "Statistics from 1995 showed that stroke is responsible for 7% of all disease mortalities. *Cardiovascular disease* is first, at 37% and cancer is second, at 28%. Accidents, including motor vehicle accidents, poisoning and violence combined accounted for only 6% of deaths and are its fourth leading cause," was my response.

"Thank you for telling us about the human cost of stroke," said a fifty-ish man who had identified himself as an economist, "but what are the economic costs?" Before starting, I had told the audience to interrupt me any time they had a question. I had learned that dialogue was an excellent way to encourage audience participation and interest; monologues are boring, even if given by charismatic people on topical subjects. Listeners tend to fall asleep after about eight minutes of a lecture, I'd been told.

"Yes," I responded, "stroke *is* very expensive. In the United States alone, the total cost for short-term hospital stays due to stroke totaled $3.8 billion in 1997. It is estimated that annual direct and indirect costs for stroke care total $40 billion. In Canada, the equivalent cost per year would be $380 million or about $12,500 for acute stroke care, and $4 billion, including direct and indirect costs—that's approximately $130,000 for stroke care for every man, woman and child."[14]

"In 1997, scientists at the National Institute of Health predicted that with continued attention to reducing the risks of stroke, using currently available therapies and developing new ones, we should be able to prevent 80% of all strokes by the end of the decade," I continued.

"But to prevent, you must first recognize. Do you know that a 1996 National Stroke Association Gallup Survey found 17% of American adults over 50 years old can't name a single stroke symptom? That's correct. Almost two out of every 10 middle-aged Americans cannot name even a single symptom of stroke. I'd like you to help me prove that Canadians can do a lot better than that. Can anyone tell me the five most common symptoms of stroke?" I asked.

"Sudden numbness or weakness of face, arm or leg, especially on one side of the body," said a lady, whom I recognized to be a patient who had recently consulted me because a CAT scan of her head requested by another physician investigating her migraine headaches reportedly showed scars suggesting past strokes. She was extremely upset by the report, especially since she was not aware of ever having had a stroke before the scan. I had informed her that CAT scans of migraine sufferers frequently showed tiny scars related to the migraines and were thus not indicators of real strokes. We then discussed what the symptoms of stroke were and I instructed her to immediately return for review if she should experience any of the symptoms. She had left my office greatly relieved.

"Wonderful! Do you recall the other four?" I encouraged her.

"Sudden confusion, trouble speaking or understanding, sudden trouble seeing in one or both eyes, sudden trouble walking, dizziness, loss of balance or coordination, and sudden severe headache with no known cause," she recited rapidly.

"Doctor, you've told us a lot about the human and economic costs of stroke, but you haven't said anything about what a stroke actually *is*. Is a stroke the same as a heart attack?" someone else asked.

In my eagerness to impress upon the audience the importance of stroke prevention, I had forgotten one of the principles of effective presentation: to first define the subject of discussion! Well, that could be easily remedied.

"A stroke, sometimes called a 'cerebrovascular accident,' is a sudden interruption of blood flow in the brain that is usually due to blockage, or a ruptured blood vessel in or leading to the brain. The interruption deprives brain tissue of essential oxygen and nutrients, and causes permanent brain damage if it continues longer than five minutes. Stroke is so named because victims appear to be suddenly struck down, as if by the 'stroke' of God's hand," I belatedly explained.

"Doctor, aren't heart attacks and strokes the same? What I mean is, both heart attack and stroke are due to the blockage of circulation. In the case of heart attack, the loss of blood flow is to the heart and in stroke the lack of blood flow is to the brain. Isn't that right?" she continued.

"You are absolutely correct. In fact, doctors now prefer to call strokes 'brain attacks' to emphasize the similarity between stroke and heart attack, the critical nature of both conditions and the immediate need for treatment," I agreed.

"If that's so, why are heart attacks painful and strokes painless?" she inquired.

Everybody in the audience knew that pain is the hallmark of heart attack. In fact, pain is universally and intuitively recognized as a symptom of disease. We all rightfully worry about heart attack as soon as we experience any chest pain. Unfortunately, stroke is different. Stroke is—discouragingly—almost always painless.

"The brain is not well supplied with pain nerve fibres and is therefore not sensitive to painful stimulation. That is why stroke is mostly painless. The heart, on the contrary, is very well supplied with nerve fibres and is therefore extremely sensitive to painful stimuli. The only pain associated with stroke is headache, which may occur with *hemorrhagic stroke* associated with bleeding in the brain. In a rare type of stroke known as *subarachnoid hemorrhage,* the headache from a ruptured *intracranial aneurysm* is particularly severe and often described as the 'worst headache' of a patient's life. The fact that most strokes are painless probably explains why more than 58% of stroke victims do not go to the emergency room until 24 hours or more after its onset.[15] Thirteen hours is the median time from stroke onset to presentation at the hospital. The other main reason for this life-threatening delay in going to the emergency is a lack of awareness of stroke symptoms, as mentioned earlier," I explained.

"Doctor, I understand what Benjamin Franklin meant when he said that time is money but recently, I've heard and read that time is brain. Can you explain?" asked a retired economist.

"Great question," I replied. "'Time is brain' means that time wasted is brain loss. Neurologists have known for a long time that the brain is very sensitive to lack of oxygen, as happens when blood flow is interrupted during a stroke. Recent studies by Dr. Jeffrey L. Saver at the Stroke Center and Department of Neurology, University of California, Los Angeles, showed that it only takes one minute for a stroke to kill nearly two million brain cells. For each hour of stroke, the brain loses at least 120 million neurons, which is equal to the number of nerve cells lost in almost 3.6 years of normal aging. The total number of neurons in the average human brain is 130 billion,[16] so every minute counts when someone is having a stroke. The longer blood flow to the brain is cut off, the greater the damage. The more brain cells that die, the more brain damage a person will sustain, resulting in disabilities or even death. The phrase 'time is brain' gained recognition when recombinant tPA was approved for the acute ischemic treatment of stroke.

"There's no doubt that stroke is a medical emergency. Immediate treatment can save people's lives and enhance their chances for successful recovery. ***Call 9-1-1 and go to the hospital immediately if you or somebody you know shows any symptom of stroke.*** Time wasted is brain loss!"

"Doctor, I thought there was no treatment for stroke—only prevention. Now you tell us to go to the hospital immediately for treatment with tPA. What is tPA?" a puzzled-looking elderly man asked.

"**Tissue plasminogen activator**—or tPA for short—is an enzyme found naturally in the body which converts *plasminogen* into the enzyme *plasmin,* which is a *thrombolytic*, an agent that dissolves blood clots. TPA is used intravenously by doctors to accelerate the dissolution of any clot blocking blood flow to the brain during a stroke. A five-year trial conducted by the United States National Institute of Neurological Disorders and Stroke (NINDS) found that carefully selected ischemic stroke patients who received the thrombolytic within three hours of the onset of stroke symptoms had a 12% absolute and 33% relative likelihood to recover from their stroke with little or no disability after three months, but with 10 times (6.4% tPA versus 0.6% placebo) the risk of serious intracranial hemorrhage than placebo patients.[17] In June 1996, tPA became the first—and is still the only—acute ischemic stroke treatment to be approved by the Federal Food and Drug Administration (FDA) in the United States.

"The Therapeutic Product directorate of Health Canada approved tPA for the similar acute treatment of ischemic stroke a year later. To be beneficial, thrombolytic or tPA therapy must be administered within three hours of stroke onset. Time is brain! To ensure the maximum benefit with the least harm, tPA must not only be administered intravenously within three hours of stroke onset but the following factors must also be excluded:

FACTORS PREVENTING tPA TREATMENT

- The onset of symptoms or the last time the patient was known to be well is greater than three hours. It is paramount that the time of stroke onset be determined as exactly as possible to fulfill the three-hour time window for tPA to be safely administered. If the patient wakes up in the morning with stroke symptoms, then the time of stroke onset is deemed to be the last time the patient was known to be well, which is usually the time that the patient went to bed or woke in the night to go to the washroom

- Rapidly improving neurological signs or minimal deficit. If the stroke symptoms are minimal or rapidly improving, then the patient may be having a *transient ischemic attack (TIA)* or "warning stroke," in which case tPA is not indicated

- Massive stroke with *obtundation, fixed-eye deviation* and complete *hemiplegia.* Coma and/or complete paralysis indicate severe stroke and increased risk of dangerous hemorrhagic complications from tPA treatment

- CAT scan evidence of *cerebral hemorrhage*

- Clinical presentation consistent with *subarachnoid hemorrhage,* even if a CAT scan is normal

- Elevated blood pressure equal to or higher than 185/110 and not treatable

- Blood glucose of less than three or more than 22 mmol/L

- Use of anticoagulants, such as *warfarin* in previous 48 hours

- Platelet count of less than 100,000

- Internal bleeding, like gastrointestinal or urinary bleeding, within past three weeks

- History of *intracranial hemorrhage, arteriovenous malformation* or *aneurysm*

- Previous stroke, major head trauma or intracranial surgery within past three months

- Recent *arterial puncture* at non-compressible site

- Major surgery within 14 days

- *Lumbar puncture* within seven days

- *Seizures* at onset of stroke

- *Myocardial infarction* within three weeks

- *Pericarditis* within three months

- Pregnancy

- Age 18 years or younger," I clarified.

"Doctor, you said that taking anticoagulants excludes you from tPA treatment. How about aspirin? Would the use of aspirin as blood thinner to prevent stroke or heart attack disqualify a person from receiving tPA for the treatment of stroke?" questioned a voice from the audience.

"No, taking aspirin to prevent stroke and heart attack does **not** exclude a person from receiving tPA for the treatment of acute ischemic stroke," I reassured the inquirer.

A retired botanist spoke up. "I know that aspirin has been proven beneficial for the secondary prevention of stroke—to avoid stroke recurrence in those who have history of cerebrovascular accidents. But I cannot tolerate aspirin because of my bleeding peptic ulcer. My doctor prescribed clopidogrel, an expensive antiplatelet medication that not only depresses my white blood cell count to dangerously low levels but also causes frequent diarrhea. My internist then prescribed *Aggrenox®*, a combination of 25 mg a.s.a. plus 200 mg. *dipyridamole*, but I developed severe migraine headaches from this platelet anti-aggregant—which was pretty expensive too, by the way. It seems like I can't tolerate any of the conventional antiplatelet agents. I remember from college that aspirin is derived from *salicin*, which is found naturally in the **white willow** plant. There are reports that white willow bark powder has the same remedial benefits as aspirin, such as prevention of stroke, but with apparently fewer side effects than the man-made compound. And it's available relatively inexpensively in 400 mg capsules in most health foods stores! I realize there is no randomized control trial proving that white willow bark prevents stroke, so I'm hesitant to rely on it for stroke prevention. I haven't used blood thinners for several months and have been lucky so far. I have had no further symptoms to suggest a recurring stroke, but then again, you've got to keep in mind the man falling off of a 100-storey building congratulating himself on the way down with, 'so far so good'! I know that it's healthier to take some kind of protection than to be completely unprotected. Can you suggest any natural blood thinners that may prevent stroke?" he asked.

I thought about it. "I should emphasize that you must be absolutely intolerant of all the standard medically recognized platelet inhibitors before trying non-phamaceutical natural blood thinners. However, the following are some natural therapies with reported antiplatelet properties:

NATURAL PLATELET INHIBITORS

- *Policosanol,* a mixture of plant alcohols most often derived from sugar cane. Clinical trials apparently found that 20 mg of policosanol daily is just as effective as 100 mg of aspirin a day [18]

- *Omega-3 fatty acids* or purified fish oil. Evidence continues to accumulate that eating 1–2 grams of omega-3 fatty acids inhibits blood clotting, thereby preventing stroke. Many specialists advise healthy individuals to consume a total of 300 to 500 mg of *docosahexaenoic acid* (DHA) and *eicosapentaenoic acid* (EPA) (combined) daily to help prevent heart disease. The American Heart Association recommends that individuals with coronary heart disease boost their omega-3 fatty acid intake to 1,000 mg a day. Most 1,000 mg fish oil capsules provide 300 mg of EPA and DHA, but some deliver as much as 600 mg. Omega-3 fatty acid supplements are routinely prescribed in Europe to treat heart attack

- *Vitamin D.* A recent trial shows the sunshine vitamin significantly reduces blood clotting in cancer patients and may therefore prevent stroke.[19] I would suggest 1,000 units daily

- Favouring foods high in *salicylates,* the natural source of aspirin, such as:
  - *Herbs and spices,* including **curry powder, cayenne pepper, ginger, paprika, thyme, cinnamon, dill, oregano** and **turmeric.**
  - *Nuts*
  - *Fruits*

- *Vitamin E (α-tocopherol,* or *alpha-tocopherol)* in 400 IU daily reputedly retards blood clotting

- *Garlic* in a daily dosage of eight grams (two to four cloves) of the raw vegetable or 600 mg of the dried herb (standardized to 1.3% *alliin* or 0.6% *allicin* yield) two to three times per day, or 14.4 grams of aged garlic extract reportedly retards blood clotting. **Onions** also have this effect but it is not as profound as with garlic
- *Ginkgo biloba,* in a dosage of 40 mg of the extract containing 24% *ginkgo heterosides* three times a day, is claimed to be an effective platelet anti-aggregant

- *Tree Ear mushroom* or *Wood Ear mushroom* (*Auricularia Polytricha*), whose name comes from the fungus' resemblance to an ear growing on a tree and is also known as *black fungus, cloud ear* and *Judas's ear*, is a native of Asia and has been a staple of **Traditional Chinese Medicine (TCM)** and cuisines for more than four centuries. Tree ear mushroom is reputed to have blood thinning properties. Chinese herbalists have been using tree ear fungus to treat heart disease and stroke for millennia. The best and most delicious technique of using wood ear fungus is as an addition to soups, stir-fries and casseroles, particularly to Asian recipes. Tree ear mushroom partners well with vegetables, grains, rice, kasha, noodles, beef, pork, poultry and seafood. The fungus is readily available fresh or dried in Chinese groceries. To reconstitute the dried mushrooms: boil for about 30 minutes or until they soften, remove from heat, allow to cool, drain and discard water. Rinse under running water after trimming the tough, fibrous portions. Add to the recipe toward the end of cooking.

"You should add these natural platelet inhibitors to a healthy lifestyle, including regular exercise, as part of your stroke prevention regimen. You must know that these natural aspirin alternatives are not a substitute for warfarin (rat poison), which is an entirely different type of blood thinner. Do not—repeat, **NOT**—adapt or mix these natural blood thinners with other heart medications, specifically anticoagulants, without first talking with your doctor."

I looked around the audience. Another hand went up.

"My name is Gene Heritage and I'm a life insurance broker. My father and two of my older brothers had strokes at an early age. My actuarialized risk for stroke is astronomically high because of my genetics. I learned from my siblings that aspirin thins blood, preventing recurrent stroke. Although I've never, ever had any symptoms of stroke, I'm afraid of suffering the number one cause of permanent disability and third cause of death because of my family history and proactively started taking a coated baby aspirin every day two years ago—just after my 49th birthday. Eight months ago, I was hospitalized for a week because of severe anemia from internal bleeding that required a blood transfusion—four units! My doctor blamed aspirin for my blood loss and I have not taken any aspirin since. Now I wonder if I even need it. Doctor, what is the evidence for or against aspirin to prevent a first stroke?"

"The short answer is that there is precious little evidence to support the use of aspirin for the prevention of a first stroke. Studies show that a.s.a. is effective in the prevention of recurrent stroke—what is known as *secondary prevention*—but that it is unlikely to be beneficial and may be even harmful because of the risk of serious internal bleeding if used to prevent a first stroke, or what is medically known as *primary prevention*. The safest and most effective primary stroke prevention strategies are quitting smoking, regular exercise, healthy diet, salt avoidance and serenity," I told him.

"Are there any natural remedies that could alleviate my genetic predisposition to stroke?" Mr. Heritage next asked.

"Yes—even though heredity has traditionally been considered the most unchangeable of the risk factors for stroke," I told him.

"Well, that's comforting. I'm greatly relieved but would like to hear more about the possibilities of offsetting inherited traits."

I told him to phone my office for an appointment to further discuss the emerging sciences of *epigenetics* and *nutrigenomics*. *(see Chapter 5).*

"Doctor, why do you keep saying 'ischemic stroke'?" another man inquired. "Is there any other type?"

"There are two major forms of stroke," I explained. "The most common type is ischemic stroke, which is a lack of blood flow due to a blockage of circulation in the brain. These blockages are responsible for about 80% of all strokes. Ischemic stroke may be *embolic*—which occurs when a blood clot (*embolus*), formed elsewhere in the body, is dislodged and travels through the bloodstream to lodge in arteries in the brain, blocking normal blood flow. Another variety of ischemic stroke occurs when a blood clot forms in the wall of arteries already damaged by high blood pressure, high cholesterol or smoking, and blocks circulation to the brain. This type is called *thrombotic* stroke. A less common variety is *hemorrhagic* stroke, which is a leakage of blood into or around the brain. Hemorrhage into or around the brain usually occurs in patients with high blood pressure, with intracranial *arteriovenous malformation*—a congenital abnormal tangle of arteries and veins that bleeds easily—or intracranial aneurysm. Hemorrhagic stroke is an absolute contraindication against the use of tPA," I concluded.

"Doctor, I've heard of a *lacunar* stroke, too—what is that?" another man wanted to know.

"*Lacunes* are tiny strokes caused by the blockage of a single deep-penetrating artery, a small artery supplying the deeper part of the brain. Lacunar strokes are often discovered on routine CAT scans of the brain. It is estimated that 25% of strokes are lacunar in type," was my answer.

"I recently heard of something called a '*whispering* stroke.' Is that the same as a lacunar stroke?" was the follow-up question.

"So-called whispering strokes are very mild, brief strokes causing either minimal or no symptoms of weakness or numbness so that they are often ignored by the victim. Although usually disregarded, an accumulation of whispering strokes can lead to permanent mental and physical impairment. As Benjamin Franklin said, 'Little strokes fell great oaks.'" I told them.

"Another kind of stroke is known as a TIA, short for *transient ischemic attack* and more commonly called a *mini* or *warning stroke*. They are caused by a temporary disturbance in the blood supply to the brain, resulting in brief neurologic dysfunction of less than 24 hours duration and usually no permanent brain damage. TIAs are also called 'warning' strokes because the risk of a major stroke is as high as 10% after one week and 20% at three months following a TIA.[a] Approximately 33% of TIAs are followed by a major stroke. Though TIAs are tiny strokes, causing only very mild or brief symptoms that usually go unnoticed or are ignored by the patient, nevertheless they can cumulatively cause permanent brain damage in the form of cognitive impairment. More alarmingly, up to 15% of TIAs go on to full blown strokes within a few short weeks of emergence.[20]

"A classic example of TIA is *amaurosis fugax* (Greek for 'fleeting darkness')—recently called *transient monocular blindness* (TMB)—a temporary loss of vision usually related to a partial or complete blockage of one of the two main arteries (the carotid arteries) in front of the neck supplying the brain. Patients usually describe *amaurosis fugax* like a curtain or a shade coming halfway down so that they cannot see the upper half of their normal field of vision in the affected eye. This 'shade effect' generally lasts for about five minutes. *Amaurosis fugax* is painless and is often associated with a *bruit* over the offending blocked carotid artery," I added.

"What is a bruit?" was the immediate follow-up question from the floor.

"A bruit is a swishing sound heard with a stethoscope, usually over a partially blocked artery. The bruit occurs because of the turbulence of circulation as blood rushes to overcome the nar-

---

a The percentage of TIAs resulting in strokes are dependent on the interval between the TIA and stroke onset.

rowing of the artery and is synchronous—in time—with your heartbeat. A bruit heard over the carotid artery usually indicates a *stenosis* (narrowing) of the artery," I explained.

Another hand went up.

"Doctor, my wife had a TIA a year ago and was told she had a carotid bruit for which she underwent extensive tests, including a carotid ultrasound that showed less than 30% blockage of the artery. Her doctor recommended that she continue on coated baby aspirin (81 mg) daily to thin her blood. Three months ago, her older sister had a similar TIA and the same doctor recommended she undergo surgery to remove the carotid stenosis within a week of her stroke. My wife and I are still puzzled as to the difference in treatment of the same condition by the same doctor, especially since they're sisters," a sixty-ish man wondered.

"Hmm. Sounds like your sister-in-law likely had an emergency *carotid endarterectomy,* a surgical procedure in which a surgeon corrects the stenosis in the artery causing the TIA. The North American Symptomatic Carotid Endarterectomy Trial (NASCET) found that endarterectomies performed by skillful surgeons[b] reduce the estimated two-year risk of stroke in symptomatic patients with between 70% to 99% carotid artery stenosis by more than 80%—a reduction from a greater than 1 in 4 chance to less than 1 in 10. In other words, at the two-year mark, endarterectomy had prevented one major stroke for every six symptomatic patients with between 70% to 99% carotid arterial stenosis.

"To determine whether or not endarterectomy is warranted, hospitals use a rating system based on need to treat (NNT). Endarterectomies have a highly cost-effective NNT number of six. To put that in perspective, the number needed to treat to prevent one heart attack in people taking the most prescribed cholesterol-lowering medication for three and one-third years

a With an operative complication rate of 5% or less,

is 100, or about 16.66 times more than endarterectomy. Symptomatic patients with less severe carotid stenosis of between 50 – 69% had a smaller benefit, with a NNT of 22 at five years. The benefit of carotid endarterectomy for symptomatic patients with 30% to 69% stenosis is therefore even less, so the operation might be considered only for good surgical risk patients who are judged to be in danger of imminent stroke. Carotid endarterectomy is not beneficial for carotid stenosis of less than 30%, even if the person is symptomatic.[21] The risk assessment of carotid endarterectomy varies with the hospital, the surgeon and the underlying disease conditions. Without seeing more medical information regarding your wife, I would suspect that tests showed her symptomatic carotid stenosis were less than 30% and so her doctor rightfully recommended her to continue taking aspirin for stroke prevention."

"I'm a health care economist and am very interested to know the total cost of a carotid endarterectomy. Obviously, if the cost of the operation is far greater than the societal loss from stroke, then the surgery might not be economically justified—even if it is extremely effective for a highly selected group of patients and done by highly specialized, experienced surgeons," the same man said.

I nodded. "You'll be pleased to know that the average total cost for the diagnostic tests, surgical procedure, hospitalization and follow-up care for a carotid endarterectomy is about $15,000. In 1990, the estimated average lifetime cost of stroke per patient in the United States was $104,000 for all stroke subtypes and $91,000 for ischemic stroke," I replied.

"So," he jumped in, "for every six operations costing $15,000 each for a total of $90,000, one stroke that costs around $100,000 is prevented, and the health care system saves more than $10,000 for each prevented stroke," the economist quickly calculated.

"And that's just the financial savings," I added. "We mustn't forget the tremendous gain in physical, emotional, psychological and mental well-being to the person saved from a stroke."

A woman who had been listening intently spoke up. "Doctor, this *amaurosis fugax* description of a warning stroke worries me. I had blurry, spotty loss of vision in half of my field of vision for about 15 to 20 minutes a couple of months ago and my ophthalmologist told me it was a migraine. I told him that I didn't even have a headache, but he still insisted it was a migraine. I used to get migraines in my twenties but have had only normal headaches easily relieved by Tylenol® since. So was he right?" asked an understandably anxious well-groomed woman who had identified herself as a schoolteacher.

I smiled at her reassuringly. "Your ophthalmologist was correct," I said. "What you experienced was an *ophthalmic migraine aura*. A classic migraine is usually preceded by blurry, spotty, wavy, zigzagging, bright, colourful visual disturbances, usually over half of the visual field of either eye and lasting about 15 to 30 minutes. This classic migraine symptom is usually followed by a headache that is generally worse on the side opposite the visual disturbance. But with an ophthalmic migraine, you experience just the visual aura but not the subsequent headache."

The lady answered my smile with a relieved one of her own.

A fit-looking woman put up her hand. "Doctor, I've had migraines for many years but never experienced any strokes and I don't have any stroke risk factors. Yet, a CAT scan of my head to evaluate my headaches reportedly showed tiny scars that the radiologist said might be related to strokes. My family doctor says not to worry and that the scars are likely due to my history of migraines rather than strokes. Who should I believe?"

I explained, "It's not uncommon to see some tiny changes in the white matter of the brain on CAT scans of migraine-sufferers that are frequently but usually erroneously reported as old strokes."

"You've told us about whispering strokes, but there's also something called a *silent* stroke too, right?" asked another.

Again I nodded. "Routine CAT scanning shows that approximately 10% of the general population has had a stroke of which they are not aware. It is likely the stroke happened when they were asleep and therefore occurred in the so-called 'silent area' of the brain. Although not felt, these silent strokes may cause problems later on, resulting in things like seizures or cognitive impairment," I informed the audience.

"Doctor, you said that strokes are all similar in that they are caused by blockages in blood circulation to the brain. Why then does it affect people differently? My father had a stroke and he lost his speech and was paralysed. But my grandfather had a stroke and he was able to speak, though he had double vision and kind of walked like he was drunk," an obviously perplexed young lady asked.

I thought about how to answer her. "The symptoms of stroke depend on the part of the brain that's damaged. Let me elaborate. The brain has three main components—the *cerebrum*, the *cerebellum* and the *brain stem*. The **cerebrum** is the largest and most developed part of the brain. It is responsible for our higher mental functions including intelligence, emotion, memory and speech. The cerebrum is divided into a right and a left hemisphere and each hemisphere is then subdivided into the *frontal, parietal, temporal* and *occipital* lobes. The left hemisphere controls most of the functions of the right side of the body and, in right-handed individuals, is where the speech centre is located so that a stroke involving the left hemisphere can cause any or all right-sided weaknesses, loss of sensation, loss of speech and loss of vision. Damage to the right cerebral hemisphere results in similar weakness, numbness and visual loss but on the left side of the body and, in left-handed individuals, also speech impairment.

"The **cerebellum** is smaller than the cerebrum and is located in the back of the brain behind the cerebrum. The cerebellum is responsible for balance and coordination. Stroke damage to the cerebellum results in a staggering gait with or without incoordination of arm and leg movement.

"The third major component of the brain is the **brain stem**, which is located underneath the cerebral hemispheres. The brain stem is where the vital centres of respiration, heart rhythm, blood pressure, wakefulness, arousal, eye movement and attention are located. The brain stem also serves as the connection between the brain and the spinal cord. Damage to the brain stem may therefore cause things like double vision, difficulty breathing, heart rate irregularity, rapid blood pressure fluctuations, sleepiness and even total body paralysis. Brain stem strokes are usually the most devastating and often leave survivors with severe permanent impairment, including that of a chronic vegetative state," I said.

"Doctor, you have spoken a lot about the blockage of circulation to the brain being the cause of ischemic strokes, but you haven't mentioned anything about what the components of circulation are," someone said.

"You're right," I apologized. "There are four arteries supplying the brain with fresh oxygenated blood. The largest are the *left* and *right internal carotid arteries*, which are branches of the common carotid arteries in the neck. After entering the cranium through the base of the skull, the internal carotid artery divides into the *anterior cerebral artery* and the *middle cerebral artery* to supply the cerebral hemispheres. The other two are smaller arteries—the *left* and *right vertebral arteries*—which are branches of the corresponding subclavian arteries and enter the cranium by way of the *foramen magnum,* or the large opening in the base of the skull where the spinal cord connects to the brain stem. Inside the cranium, which houses the brain, the vertebral arteries fuse to form the *basilar artery,* which then divides into the *posterior cerebral arteries* that supply fresh oxygenated blood to the back part of the cerebral hemispheres, brain stem and cerebellum. The internal carotid arteries are interconnected via the *anterior communicating artery* and with the basilar artery via the *posterior communicating arteries* to form the *Circle of Willis,* named after Dr. Thomas Willis, the famous English physician who first described this very important vascular formation. The Circle of Willis provides an alternative route of bypassing a blockage in one of main cerebral arteries, allowing blood to continue flowing to tissues that would otherwise become ischemic," I described.

A middle-aged lady then spoke, doing her best to control her emotions. "My husband had a stroke six months ago. He is now walking with the aid of a cane but he has become increasingly forgetful. He can't remember anything. He forgets everything, especially recent events. Yesterday, I told him I was attending this meeting today. This morning, when I was getting dressed to come here, he asked where I was going and I told him again. A few minutes later, he again asked where I was going and I repeated that I was coming here. Then, just as I was leaving, he again asked where I was going." She paused to collect herself. "This has been going on since shortly after his stroke. He was never like this before and nobody in his family has memory problems. I was worried that he was developing Alzheimer's disease so I talked to his family doctor about it. The doctor said that my husband likely has *vascular dementia*, which I understand is a type of dementia that results from strokes and not Alzheimer's disease. His family doctor also said that vascular dementia can even develop in people who have no history of a stroke but who just have risk factors for a stroke. Now I'm worried that I might develop vascular dementia even though I've never have a stroke. Doctor, please tell us the risk factors for stroke and how we can avoid or minimize them."

I was glad she'd asked; everyone needs this information. "The risk factors are genetic traits and lifestyle habits that increase the risk of disease; in this case, the danger of stroke and, as you mentioned, vascular dementia," I told her. "Vascular dementia used to be called *multi-infarct dementia*, which, as the name implies, is dementia associated with stroke. However, recent studies are convincing doctors that even having stroke risk factors may lead to cognitive decline—even in the absence of stroke history." I could see people in the audience getting ready to take notes. Obviously the idea of dementia based on risk factors alone was a troublesome one.

I continued. "The risk factors for stroke are customarily divided into uncontrollables and controllables. Factors long believed to be uncontrollable may now evidently be partly modifiable by healthy lifestyle, and dietary and environmental changes that we'll discuss later.

"UNCONTROLLABLE" STROKE RISK FACTORS

- **Age**: the chance of having a stroke approximately doubles for each decade of life after age 55
- **Heredity**: the risk of stroke is greater if there is a family history of stroke
- **Race**: people of African descent have a much higher risk of death from a stroke than Caucasians do. This is partly because they have higher risks of high blood pressure, diabetes and obesity
- **Gender**: stroke is more common in men than in women
- **Prior stroke, TIA or heart attack**: the risk of stroke for someone who has already had one is many times that of a person who has not. For example, having had a transient ischemic attack (TIA) or warning stroke increases your risk of suffering a major stroke by a factor of 10.

"The following 'controllable' stroke risk factors are change-able, usually with medications, though I will also tell you about natural, non-pharmaceutical modifications that are evidently equally effective and are without the side effects of drugs.

"CONTROLLABLE" STROKE RISK FACTORS

- **High blood pressure** is the most important controllable risk factor for stroke
- **Cigarette smoking** is probably the most difficult correctable risk factor for stroke
- **Oral contraceptives** greatly increase stroke risk, especially in smokers who also suffer from migraines
- **Diabetes mellitus**
- **Heart disease,** particularly *coronary insufficiency* and *atrial fibrillation*
- **High blood cholesterol**
- **Unhealthy diets** that are high in saturated fat, trans-fat, cholesterol, salt, calories and low in fibre
- **Physical inactivity**
- **Obesity**
- **Alcohol abuse** is associated with higher stroke risk
- **Drug abuse**, including addiction to cocaine, amphetamines and heroin, has been associated with an increased risk of stroke
- **Psychological stress**, like anxiety, fear, depression, anger and hatred, are increasingly being recognized as risk factors for stroke
- **Infection** and **inflammation** are high risk factors for stroke
- **Vitamin D deficiency** has been shown to be a possible independent risk factor for stroke.[22]

"Most of these stroke risk factors have also been associated with vascular dementia, but increasing age, history of stroke, high blood pressure and diabetes are the strongest ones. Later on, I'll discuss some natural strategies to modify, prevent, avoid or minimize the most damaging of them." The easiest, safest, cheapest and probably most effective measures to prevent dementia are to:

DEMENTIA PREVENTION

- Socialize, dance or play cards,
- Exercise, walk for about 30 minutes three to four times a week
- Eat lots of small oily fish, such as sardines.

I nodded at a middle-aged man with his hand up.

"Doctor, my 90-year-old mother is still living independently in her own home on the farm. She had two younger sisters, both of whom lived in heavily industrialized cities down East and both of whom died of stroke in their early sixties from what my mother describes as 'polluted air' or 'pollution poisoning.' My mother claims that her personal good health is primarily due to the clean, fresh, rural air she's breathed all her life. Is this just her superstition or is there scientific proof to substantiate her belief that polluted air is a risk factor for stroke?"

"That's a great question. Yes, your mother is absolutely correct. There *is* cumulative evidence that ambient air pollution is a modifiable risk factor for stroke. Dr. Chun-Yuh Yang and co-investigators at the Kaohsiung Medical University in Taiwan found an association between exposure to increasing levels of ambient air pollutants and hospital admissions for stroke, particularly on warm days.[23]

"In another analysis of outdoor air pollution and stroke data in Sheffield, England, Dr. Ravi Maheswaran and colleagues discovered that an 11% increase of stroke mortality is attributable to outdoor air pollution.[24] The association of stroke and air pollution may be explained by the findings of Nino Kuenzil, vice director of the Swiss Tropical and Public Institute and fellow researchers from the University of Southern California Artherosclerosis Research Unit, who found that the progression of atherosclerosis was two times faster among the 1,483 participants who live within 100 metres of Los Angeles highways, compared to their peers who live further away.[25] So your mother has compelling scientific support for her 'superstition' that polluted air is a modifiable risk factor for stroke. It is modifiable because you can avoid the dangers of air pollution by living in cleaner ambient air areas and staying indoors or wearing a *N95 mask* if you must venture outside on high smog days," I acknowledged.

"Dr. Veloso, I understand that *hypertension* or high blood pressure is the most important modifiable risk factor for stroke, but what about *prehypertension*?" asked another listener.

I was already nodding. "Blood pressure is the force exerted on your artery walls as blood flows through your body. Slightly elevated blood pressure is known as **prehypertension**. Left untreated, prehypertension is likely to progress to definite high blood pressure. Both prehypertension and high blood pressure increase your risk of heart attack, stroke and heart failure," I explained and continued, "A blood pressure reading has two numbers. The first, or upper, number measures the pressure in your arteries when your heart beats (*systolic pressure*). The second, or lower, number measures the pressure in your arteries between beats (*diastolic pressure*). **Normal blood pressure** is below 120 systolic/80 diastolic, as measured in millimetres of mercury (mm Hg).

"**Prehypertension** is a systolic pressure from 120 to 139 or a diastolic pressure from 80 to 89. When prehypertension was defined as a new category of blood pressure in 2003, many people who thought they had normal blood pressure were surprised to learn that their blood pressure was now considered elevated. Why the new category? To reinforce the health risks of even *slightly* elevated blood pressure. You can't see or feel prehypertension, but there's plenty you can do about it. Weight loss, exercise and other healthy lifestyle changes can often control prehypertension—and set the stage for a lifetime of better health. Prehypertension doesn't cause symptoms. In fact, even advanced high blood pressure may not cause symptoms. The only way to detect prehypertension is to keep track of your blood pressure readings. Have your blood pressure checked at each doctor's visit or check it yourself at home with a home blood pressure monitoring device. But be aware that blood pressure measurements from a device in a pharmacy or other public location may not be accurate if the cuff isn't the right size for you or if the device hasn't been serviced regularly," I said.

"What causes prehypertension?" she then asked.

"Any factor that increases pressure against artery walls:

CAUSES OF PREHYPERTENSION

- Family history of high blood pressure
- Sedentary lifestyle
- Diet high in sodium or low in potassium
- Cigarette smoking
- Alcohol abuse
- Obesity
- A narrowing of the arteries and/or an increase in blood volume from whatever cause
- Certain medical conditions such as sleep apnea, kidney and adrenal diseases
- Some medications, like birth control pills, cold remedies and decongestants
- Illegal drugs, particularly cocaine and amphetamines

but more often high blood pressure creeps up silently over many years without a specific identifiable cause," I replied.

"So when should I get tested for prehypertension," asked the now understandably anxious woman.

"You should have a blood pressure reading at least every two years and more frequently if the measurements tend to be higher or lower than the normal of 120/80. Higher blood pressure readings are classified as:

- **Prehypertension**: 120/80 to 139/89
- **Stage 1 hypertension**: 140/90 to 159/99
- **Stage 2 hypertension**: 160/100 or higher

"Because blood pressure tends to fluctuate, a diagnosis of prehypertension is based on the average of two or more blood pressure readings taken on separate occasions in a consistent manner.

"In addition to the increased risk of heart attack, stroke and heart failure, prehypertension can also damage your organs. And it tends to get worse over time. Within four years of being diagnosed with prehypertension, nearly one in three adults ages 35 to 64 and nearly one in two adults age 65 or older progresses to definite high blood pressure, according to the American Heart Association.[26]

"As your blood pressure increases, so does your risk of cardiovascular disease. That's why it's so important to control prehypertension," I cautioned.

"So, how *do* you control prehypertension?" queried the lady.

"The key is a commitment to healthy lifestyle changes," I informed her.

"What about fruit and vegetables? I've been hearing that a diet high in fruit and vegetables prevents stroke. Is there any scientific basis for that recommendation?" asked an elderly lady.

"There are numerous studies supporting the advice that a diet rich in fruit and vegetables prevents stroke, but I will just cite the research of F.J. He and C.A. Nowson who conducted a meta-analysis of eight studies regarding the relationship between fruit and vegetable consumption and risk of stroke that included 257,551 individuals followed for an average of 13 years. They found that those who ate five or more servings of fruit and vegetables daily reduced the risk of suffering a stroke by up to 26% compared to participants who consumed three or less servings a day, with the greatest reduction attributed to the higher number of servings," I told her.[27]

"Doctor, we've all heard that the risks for stroke are traditionally based on the unchangeable factors of age, gender, race and heredity and the changeable problems of hypertension, cigarette smoking, past history of stroke and diabetes, but recently I've also heard that blood abnormalities such as *C-reactive protein* and *homocysteinemia* are also stroke risk factors. Is that your understanding?" asked a retired biology teacher.

"Yes," I said. "**C-reactive protein (CRP)** is a protein produced by the body in response to inflammation of any kind, including traumatic injury, infection, arthritis and malignancy. In the Framingham Study of 591 men and 871 women with an average age of 69.7 years followed over 14 years, Dr. Philip Wolf and his associates from the Boston University School of Medicine found that individuals with the highest percentage of C-reactive protein in their blood had two times the risk of suffering a stroke compared to their peers with the lowest level of C-reactive protein.[28] Several other studies have confirmed that a high blood level of C-reactive protein is an independent risk factor for stroke.

"**Homocysteine** is an amino acid normally present in blood and is produced from the metabolism of *methionine,* an essential amino acid. A high level of homocysteine is associated with an increased incidence of stroke, but unfortunately, efforts to lower homocysteine levels with high doses of vitamins including *folic acid, pyridoxine* and *cobalamin*, which normally metabolize homocysteine, have not been shown to reduce that risk," I replied.

"What about drinking alcohol?" asked another. "I've heard both recommendations for and condemnations against alcohol consumption. Does having the occasional alcoholic beverage have anything to do with stroke prevention?" questioned a voice from the back of the room.

"Alcohol is the perfect example of Mark Twain's saying, 'Water, taken in moderation, cannot hurt anybody,' and Terence's dictum, 'Moderation in all things.' Alcohol in small daily quantities such as one to two ounces of whiskey or its equivalent of two beers or two standard eight-ounce glasses of wine—preferably red—prevents stroke and heart attacks, but more than the recommended two ounces a day is harmful and can result in serious medical problems, including liver damage, increased risk for heart attack and stroke, inflammation of the stomach or pancreas, high blood pressure, cancers and seizures.[29] I would strongly caution anyone from exceeding the recommended two ounces of alcohol daily—and most definitely not before driving or while participating in any activity that requires your full attention and concentration," I emphasized.

And then came the comment that had surprised me most and made me remember Mrs. Patience now, two weeks later, when her husband had been admitted to the emergency room I was rapidly nearing.

"Dr. Veloso, I understand that tPA can be an effective treatment for stroke under certain conditions, but can you tell us about snake venom as a possible treatment option?" she'd asked.

There had been several raised eyebrows in the crowd and I myself had been astonished by her question. This was a meeting for the general public; the audience was not expected to know state-of-the-art medical research! Very few doctors, including specialists, knew about the study of snake poison as a treatment for acute ischemic stroke. I was very curious as to how a non-health care professional grandmotherly-type in a prairie city had learned that snake venom was being tested for the treatment of stroke.

So I said, "Before I answer your remarkable inquiry, may I ask how you know about snake venom as a potential stroke treatment?"

Mrs. Patience had smiled and said, "My son is a post-graduate student in pharmacology. He just returned from China where he was studying herbs used in traditional Chinese medicine and he told me that the Chinese are using a snake poison in the treatment of stroke. He said that they have had some success with the viper venom. I don't think he was joking," she said.

I was amazed by how small a world it is that brand-new research like this could be known already. The hospital I worked at had just completed participation in a clinical research trial regarding *ancrod*, the venom of the Malayan pit viper, and a potent natural anticoagulant. Ancrod works by reducing blood levels of *fibrinogen*, a critical agent in blood clotting, thereby breaking down existing blood clots and preventing new ones from forming, thinning out the blood so that circulation to the brain is improved.

Tissue plasminogen activator, tPA, had been approved by Health Canada for the treatment of acute ischemic stroke within three hours of onset. The snake venom research had studied whether the poison might double the time window from three to six hours during which stroke victims could be safely treated. If the time window for effective, safe blood clot-buster treatment doubled from three to six hours, the number of stroke victims treated could expand from the current three to possibly more than 40 out of a hundred, more than 13 times the current number we were able to treat. The savings in lives and money would be immense. The pivotal phase of the ancrod research had been completed and I'd just found out the study was, unfortunately, negative.

"Your son wasn't pulling your leg," I had responded. "We participated in an acute stroke study using the venom of the Malayan pit viper, generically known as ancrod. Ancrod was discovered when doctors found that the blood of people who had been bitten by the Malayan pit viper did not clot normally for several days afterward. I believe the Chinese are studying the snake venom of the *Southern Anhui Agkistrodon acutus*, which also dissolves blood clots, and that they are having some success with it," I had added.

Yes, I definitely remembered Prudence Patience and her knowledge of snake venom as a treatment for acute stroke. Now I would have to see if I could help her husband, I thought as I entered the hospital at a run.

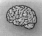

The Five Symptoms of Stroke

- Sudden numbness or weakness of the face, arm or leg, especially on one side of the body
- Sudden confusion or trouble speaking or understanding speech
- Sudden trouble seeing in one or both eyes
- Sudden trouble walking, dizziness or loss of balance or coordination
- Sudden severe headache with no known cause.

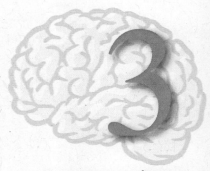

time is brain

*"Natural forces within us
are the true healers of disease."*

~ Hippocrates

"Nature, time and patience are the three great physicians."

~ Bulgarian Proverb

"Where is Mr. Patience?" I asked as soon as I arrived in the emergency room.

"He was taken immediately to Radiology for a CT scan of his head," Florence Strokeller, the stroke nurse replied.

"Did you give him the informed consent form for tPA treatment to read and sign?" I asked.

"Yes, Dr. Veloso, but Mr. Patience said that he doesn't understand the information on the form and wants us to contact his son Patrick in Vancouver for consent to use tPA to treat his stroke," Florence said.

The patient information and consent form the stroke nurse gave to Mr. Patience looked like this:

PATIENT INFORMATION AND CONSENT FORM
FOR tPA ADMINISTRATION

You have experienced a brain attack. It is also called a stroke, a brain infarction, an ischemic stroke or a cerebrovascular accident. The kind of stroke you have experienced is caused by a blood clot that is blocking the blood supply to your brain. Because of this clot, a portion of your brain is exposed to permanent damage. Recent research supported by treatment experience tells us that if we can dissolve the clot within three hours of the beginning of the stroke, we may be able to reduce the amount of damage to your brain that may be caused by this clot.

Your doctors are prepared to use a medication to help minimize this damage. It is called tPA or recombinant tissue plasminogen activator. This drug, which must be given through a vein, may dissolve the clot. TPA is a natural substance normally produced by the body. However, treatment with this drug will result in large amounts of this substance circulating in your body during the time the drug is actually being given to you. It is administered over a one-hour period of time.

Before the discovery of this drug, patients who suffered a stroke had only a one-in-five chance of full recovery of all neurologic functions. With tPA, there is an increased chance you will recover nearly completely (approximately a 31% chance). A full recovery can also occur.

The use of this drug in stroke patients is new but is supported by the results of a large study conducted by the United States government's National Institutes of Health. This is the only Health Protection Branch (HPB) of Health and Welfare Canada approved treatment currently proven effective in limiting the brain damage from a stroke.

Although it is the best treatment recommended, tPA is not without risk. There is a 6% chance that it will cause bleeding in the brain. Patients with strokes may die as a result of this treatment. This drug should not be administered later than three hours from the time your stroke symptoms began. The drug will maximize the chance that your brain will be able to fully recover if the clot is dissolved.

Even with the precautions your doctors are taking, there is no guarantee that serious bleeding or death will not occur. This drug can also cause bleeding in other parts of the body.

WITH YOUR SIGNATURE, YOU ARE INDICATING THAT YOU FULLY UNDERSTAND THIS TREATMENT, ITS POSSIBLE BENEFITS AND RISKS AND THAT YOU AGREE TO RECEIVE THE DRUG tPA.

Patient's name: _____

Signature of Patient,
Significant Other or Representative:

_____

Date: _____

If you are not the patient, please print your name and your relationship to the patient, below

---

Witness (Optional)   *Print Name Signature   Date*

Physician's Name   *Signature   Date*

NOTE: *This form to be completed in addition to a regular consent for treatment/procedure.*[a]

"Did Mr. Patience give you his son's telephone number?" I asked, glancing at the clock and noting that it was already 8:15 a.m. The window for tPA treatment was rapidly narrowing!

"He doesn't remember it, but Mrs. Patience said that she always carries her address book with her. You may be able to get their son's telephone number from her," the stroke nurse told me.

"Where is she?" I asked urgently.

"In the waiting room," was the immediate answer.

I found Mrs. Patience sobbing in a corner chair.

"Thank you for coming so quickly, Dr. Veloso. I remembered what you told us in your talk about calling 9-1-1 without delay so tPA treatment would be possible. I called as soon as I realized that Victor was having a stroke. He suddenly couldn't move his left side and I remembered that sudden weakness or numbness, especially of one side of the body, is one of the main symptoms of a stroke. I hope Victor arrived in time for tPA," she said, wiping the tears from her face.

---

a When tPA was first approved for the treatment of acute stroke, the Canadian Stroke Consortium recommended that the patient sign a consent form to accept the treatment because of the risks of serious bleeding from the blood clot-busting medication. In retrospect, I agree that this consent form was difficult for non-health care professionals to understand, especially someone who has just suffered a stroke. Most hospitals have now dispensed with this additional consent form before giving tPA to stroke patients, but it outlines the debate between the risks (6% chance of serious, potentially fatal brain bleeding) versus the benefits (31% probability of improved outcome) in the treatment of acute stroke.

Whether Mr. Patience had arrived in time for tPA or not depended on the time his stroke had started. TPA had to be administered within three hours of stroke onset. I looked at my watch again. It was now 8:20 a.m.

"When did he first notice he couldn't move on his left side?" I asked.

"Early this morning," she replied.

"Could you be more precise? It is crucial that I know the exact time of stroke onset to determine if your husband can benefit from tPA without undue risk of serious hemorrhage from the blood clot-busting treatment."

I urged Mrs. Patience to pinpoint the onset of her husband's stroke accurately and asked what time he customarily woke in the morning and whether his left side was already weak when he woke up. If Mr. Patience had woken with symptoms of stroke, then the time of onset would be considered to be the last time he was known to be well. If he had gone to bed at 11:00 p.m. the night before and felt well at that time, then his stroke would be deemed to have occurred at that time. If he woke at 3:00 a.m. and was able to, for example, use the washroom and return to bed on his own without assistance and then woke up later—at, say, 7:00 a.m.—with symptoms of stroke, then his stroke would be deemed to have occurred at 3:00 a.m. If a person wakes up with symptoms of a stroke, the time of onset is the last time that the individual was known to be well.

After thinking about it, Mrs. Patience exclaimed, "Victor's stroke must have happened at exactly 7:00 a.m.!"

"Are you sure? How can you be so precise?" I asked, hoping Mrs. Patience would have a solid reason to believe that her husband's stroke had occurred only an hour and twenty minutes earlier, which would leave us with an hour and forty minutes to complete all the procedures required to administer the emergency tPA treatment.

"I know it happened at exactly 7:00 a.m. because Victor listens to the CBC national news after breakfast. He was lighting up his third cigarette of the day on his way to the sofa in front of the TV when the coffee cup he was carrying in his left hand fell to the floor.

"It was the smash of the coffee cup that alarmed me. When I looked around, Victor was lying on the floor unable to move his left side and the news was just coming on. That's how I know that it was exactly 7:00 a.m. I called 9-1-1 immediately and left a message with his family doctor afterwards, as you told us we should. The ambulance got there in about 15 minutes and took him to the hospital right away. Oh, if only Victor had been able to quit smoking, he probably could've avoided this! Heaven knows how many times he's struggled to quit. Smoking is a horrible addiction." She dabbed at her eyes again.

I glanced at my watch once more. 8:30 a.m. Only 90 minutes left to safely administer tPA to Mr. Patience.

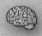

Call 9-1-1 Immediately!

Remember! Time is brain. If you or someone you know is experiencing any symptoms of a stroke, **DO NOT WAIT**. TPA is an effective therapy for stroke that must be administered at a hospital, but the treatment loses its effectiveness and becomes more dangerous if not given within the first three hours after stroke symptoms appear. Act immediately—prompt action is critical. Every minute counts!

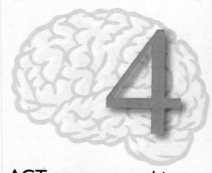

ACT to stop smoking

Acknowledge tobacco addiction
Commit to cigarette cessation
Terminate smoking tenaciously

"Sooner or later, everyone stops smoking."

~ ANONYMOUS

Victor Patience had been listening to the CBC national news after breakfast and was lighting up his third cigarette of the day when the coffee cup he was carrying in his left hand fell to the floor. He had suffered a massive stroke and now his wife wondered if his smoking had anything to do with it.

People often think of lung cancer as the main reason to stop smoking. But it is also a leading cause of stroke.

"Your brother-in-law is calling long-distance from West Virginia. He says it's an emergency," my secretary interrupted me as I concentrated on calculating the blood pressure of an elderly lady referred from the emergency room for evaluation of possible stroke. She had woken up that morning with left-sided weakness and numbness. I looked at the clock. It was 8:30 a.m.

West Virginia? It must be Ronald.

My wife is sixth in a family with 12 siblings. Son number seven is Ronald, who is a year younger than my wife. Ron had studied abroad and had not only earned a Bachelor of Arts degree but also learned to smoke. He had eventually become a cardiologist and had been practising for about 20 years when I received his urgent call. "Hi Ron. What's happened?"

"I wanted you to know I'm undergoing emergency open heart surgery tonight," he said. "My cardiovascular surgeon says that I have to stop smoking. He says that he won't operate on me unless I promise to quit."

I had heard similar words from patients many times over the years but it was still a shock to hear them uttered by a family member, especially one who was himself a heart specialist. Ron explained that he had collapsed while seeing a patient in his office that morning and was rushed to the nearest hospital where he was diagnosed as having had an acute heart attack. Ron was the only one in his family who smoked. His father and mother never smoked, and nor did any of his 11 siblings. Ron was now also the only member of his family to have suffered a heart attack. There was no trace of heart disease in the rest of the family. Growing up, they all ate the same food, drank the same water, breathed the same air, enjoyed the same sports, etc.[a]

"You know," Ron continued. I've tried to quit many times but

---

a   This type of proof is known as "anecdotal" and is not credible in today's practice of evidence-based medicine. To be acceptable to modern medical science, the evidence must be derived from randomized double-blind placebo control research. But how would you double-blind smoking? Can you imagine anybody agreeing to participate in a trial where he has a 50/50 chance of being selected to smoke or not to smoke one to two packs of cigarettes every day for 10 years? Also, is it ethical to expose anyone to cigarettes knowing that smoking may be harmful? This kind of research will never be done. Now you see how my good friend Joe—who claimed that quitting smoking was a piece of cake since he has done it hundreds of times—can justifiably state that "there is no convincing scientific evidence that smoking is harmful to me or to others."

I always go back to it. I'm just like the guy who boasted that quitting smoking is easy since he has done it hundreds of times. *You* used to be a two-pack a day smoker, Felix. How did you stop smoking?"

I had been a third-year medical student with a two-pack a day habit in 1964 when I heard over the radio one morning that the United States' Surgeon General said that cigarette smoking caused lung cancer. In class that day, I kept thinking about the reported link between an incurable disease and smoking. *A fine doctor you're going to be!* I thought to myself. *Here you are, learning how to prevent and treat diseases in others while risking the very real danger of a self-inflicted fatal illness!*

In bed that night, while stubbing out my customary last cigarette before lights out, I decided to stop smoking. But how? Needless to say, I did not sleep well.

The next day in class, the professor was lecturing on public health when I suddenly remembered his last lesson. He'd quoted from the Gospel of St. Luke: "Physician, heal thyself."[30]

So, I would cure myself of this sickness. Again, how? Then I recalled the last two lines of "Invictus": "I am the master of my fate; I am the captain of my soul."[31] I decided to psych myself into stopping smoking by repeating to myself that I would not let an inanimate stick of tobacco control my life. *I am a man. A cigarette is just a roll of dried leaves. Who is stronger? Are you a man or a mouse?* I asked myself that many times every day. The answer was always, *I am the captain of my soul; I am the master of my fate.*

After a month of this self-hypnosis, I put out my final bedtime cigarette with the resolution that the next morning would be the first day of the rest of my smoke-free life. The next few days were pure torture. I was either chewing gum or toothpicks or biting my fingernails—all the while casting covetous glances at the remaining half pack of cigarettes that I purposely carried in my shirt pocket just to prove that I would not yield to temptation. Three or four weeks later, I knew that I was well on my way to recovery when I noticed that my fingernails were growing back.

"Have a cigarette," a classmate said to me at a New Year's Eve party.

"No, thank you. I don't smoke," I proudly replied.

"Don't smoke? Come-on, this is New Year's Eve! Aren't you a real macho man? Remember the Marlboro Man."

It was near midnight. I had had a few beers. It had been more than a year since I'd stopped smoking. Surely I was cured of the addiction. There should be no harm in proving to my classmate that I was "a real macho man." We puffed on Marlboros as we welcomed the New Year, the smoke from our cigarettes lost in the hazy fumes of exploding firecrackers. The very first thing I did after waking up at noon on New Year's Day was to go all over town searching for an open store to buy cigarettes.

Five years later, I was puffing on a Chesterfield cigarette in bed at home, recovering from a bad flu, when I had a bad paroxysm of coughing. I was a full-fledged physician, having smoked through the rest of my undergraduate years, internship and my final year of residency. I slowly removed the stick of tobacco from my lips. I stared at it for the longest time while repeating, "Physician, heal thyself." Then I deliberately put out the hateful cigarette and flushed the remainder of the pack down the toilet where it belonged. Even now, 40 years later, I still have nightmares of having started smoking again.

And the tobacco industry says that cigarette smoking is not addictive!

I thought of a conversation I'd had with Joe, a good friend of mine and a long-time smoker, 15 years ago.

"My $12,000 hot steam room … *(cough, cough, cough)* … is finished. The brochure from the manufacturer says the hot steam will stop my coughing … *(cough, cough, cough)*," Joe proudly told me between cigarettes puffs during one of our customary Saturday night dinners in a smoke-filled Chinese restaurant. He had then been smoking for 45—and coughing for 30—of his 60 years.

Once, when I was trying for the umpteenth time to convince him to stop smoking, Joe had said, "Just watch me" and deliberately lit a second cigarette to puff alongside the first already half-smoked one.

I had asked Joe at dinner just the previous Saturday (we still dined at the same Chinese restaurant, though it was a non-smoking venue now) how he was doing with his $12,000 hot steam room.

"Great ... *(cough, cough, cough)* ... best money I ever invested. Can't you hear? ... *(cough, cough, cough)* ... I'm coughing much less now ... *(cough, cough, cough)* ... ."

This is the same good friend who claims, "There is no convincing scientific evidence smoking is harmful." To paraphrase Abraham Lincoln, *You can convince some people all the time, you can convince all people some of the time, but you cannot convince some people anytime.*

Needless to say, Joe, now 75, is still smoking.

"Is my blood pressure high?" a 64-year-old patient had asked anxiously after I completed her regular six-month examination following a minor stroke she had suffered three years earlier. It was a cold December day and I can still picture the sun-dogs visible through the frosted windows of my office.

Her stroke had been characterized by a sudden loss of memory lasting for about 12 hours and had been diagnosed as *transient global amnesia* due to lack of blood flow to the temporal lobe, the memory centre of the brain.

"I am sorry, but it is a bit on the high side," I said, trying not to alarm her unduly.

"How high? Is it higher than last winter?" She was not reassured.

"Only 186 over 94" I said calmly.

"186 over 94! But my blood pressure was normal when I saw you last June. I'm diligent about avoiding salt and exercising regularly. My lifestyle isn't any different. So how come my blood pressure is high in winter and normal in summer?"

I thought about it. "*Your* routine might be the same throughout the year but what about your husband's? Does he change his smoking habits with the seasons?" I knew that her husband smoked about one and a half packs of cigarettes a day.

"He smokes outside when the weather is nice, but I allow him to smoke inside the house on cold winter days. Why?"

"Well, we know that cigarette smoke can elevate blood pressure. We know that you do not smoke. We know that your husband smokes in your tightly insulated house on cold winter days. We also know that your blood pressure is elevated only in winter. I suspect that you're a victim of secondhand smoke. Do you mind if I talk to your husband about this problem?"

She readily agreed and I brought him into the office and explained my theory to him.

"So I'm responsible for my wife's high blood pressure? I can't believe it—I'm so sorry!" he said to her. Turning to me he added, "Do you think that maybe my smoking was also to blame for her stroke?" he asked. "I'll do anything to help her get better," he ended.

"I'm afraid that your smoking *is* probably responsible for her high blood pressure in winter and more than likely contributed to her stroke three years ago. I say 'winter' because the rest of the year you smoke outside and your wife is not exposed to as much secondhand smoke. This is the only circumstance that explains your wife's seasonal high blood pressure. We do have evidence that secondhand smoke is as harmful as firsthand smoke, and might be even more so."

Exposure to smoke, whether first- or secondhand, causes *platelets* (the blood cells that cause clotting) to become stickier within 30 minutes of exposure, leading to the blockage of blood vessels supplying the brain and resulting in stroke or brain attack. Worldwide, smoking tobacco accounts for 5 million premature deaths, making it the number one killer of the estimated 7 million people dead of substance abuse each year (a rate of 110 per 100,000 versus a murder rate of about 8 per 100,000). Alcohol is second, being responsible for almost 2 million deaths. In contrast, illegal drug use accounts for about 220,000 fatalities or about 3% of all drug-related deaths. If all of this is still not convincing, then think about studies that show a lifetime of smoking generally shortens your lifespan by 10 years.[32]

I told him about a city whose population of 70,000 banned indoor smoking in public places in June 2002. The heart attack rate immediately declined and, after six months, there were 58% fewer heart attacks in people living within the city limits, but no decrease for people living outside of the city where there was no similar ban.[33] When the tobacco industry succeeded in lobbying the legislature to abolish the no smoking ban, the number of heart attacks in the city immediately climbed and was back to normal within a few months. Another study in a neighbouring municipality found a 41% drop in the rate of hospitalization for heart attack three years after a ban on workplace smoking took effect. The same research shows that secondhand smoke caused an estimated 46,000 deaths from heart attack per year among non-smokers in the United States. There is also at least one study that showed that spouses exposed to secondhand smoke have about twice the risk of suffering a stroke, and other research suggests that secondhand smoke is as harmful as firsthand smoke.[34]

"I want to stop smoking but how can I do it? Dr. Veloso, please help me," said the visibly distraught man.

"You have already acknowledged your cigarette addiction—that's the most important step. You must now make up your mind to stop smoking. You must be determined. You must persevere! Repeat to yourself several times each day: **I am the cap-**

tain of my soul. I am the master of my fate. I absolutely will not let a few stinky tobacco leaves control me or my loved ones' lives.** You must not have any doubt whatsoever that you can and will stop smoking. You must tell yourself several times every day that you have stopped smoking. You must be proud to be some-one who controls his own destiny. You must remember the great American philosopher Henry David Thoreau, who said, 'What a man thinks of himself, that is which determines, or rather indi-cates, his fate.'[35] Then you will undoubtedly stop smoking."

I gave him a pamphlet, reproduced below, titled "ACT to Stop Smoking" that outlines the risks of smoking and benefits of stopping, as well as helpful strategies to combat tobacco ad-diction.

Acknowledge Tobacco Addiction

The first step is to recognize that smoking tobacco is an addic-tion, not just a bad habit. It is an addiction, period. Admit to yourself that you are an addict. Remind yourself that smokers typically die 13 to 14 years earlier than non-smokers. Accept the fact that there is irrefutable medical evidence that smok-ing cigarettes is related to more than two dozen diseases. It has negative effects on nearly every organ of the body and reduces overall health. Smoking tobacco remains the leading cause of preventable death and has negative health impacts on people of all ages: unborn babies, infants, children, adolescents, adults and seniors.

SERIOUS HEALTH PROBLEMS CAUSED BY SMOKING

- **Cancer.** The most notorious is lung cancer, which is the leading cause of death due to cancer in Canada. Smoking tobacco is the singlemost important, preventable cause of lung cancer, accounting for 85% of all new cases of lung cancer in Canada. Less well known but equally deadly malignancies related to smoking include cancer of the mouth, throat, larynx and esophagus. Studies also indicate that smoking is a contributing cause of leukemia and cancers of the bladder, stomach, kidney and pancreas.

- **Respiratory diseases.** The respiratory diseases associated with smoking include Chronic Obstructive Pulmonary Disease (COPD), emphysema, chronic bronchitis and asthmatic bronchitis.

- **Cardio-cerebrovascular diseases.** These are diseases and injuries of blood vessels of the body, particularly of the heart, causing heart attack, and of the brain, causing stroke. Cigarette smoking is a well- recognized risk factor of stroke. The risk of stroke is approximately 50% higher in smokers than in non-smokers. The risk increases with the number of cigarettes smoked per day. Smokers who consume more than 25 cigarettes daily have the highest risk of a stroke. In 1996 alone, approximately 2,500 Canadians died of smoking-related strokes.

Stopping smoking reduces the risk of stroke by approximately 50% within one year and to normal levels (comparable to those of people who have never smoked) within five years. If all of this is still not convincing enough that smoking is damaging, then perhaps the fact that smoking has also been linked to erectile dysfunction will encourage smokers to conquer their addiction.

Quitting can have immediate as well as long-term benefits. Quitting at age 65 or older can reduce by nearly 50% the risk of dying of a smoking-related disease. On the other hand, former smokers have the same stroke risk as non-smokers five to 15 years after quitting.[36] Acknowledge that your secondhand smoke exposes your loved ones to the same degree of risk of developing serious diseases, particularly stroke. Researchers found that spouses exposed to secondhand smoke are approximately two times more at risk of developing strokes compared to spouses of non-smokers.

Commit to Cigarette Cessation

You must be determined to stop smoking. You must be merciless. Do not let tobacco take you prisoner. There are no exceptions. Once you decide to stop, you must vanquish your addiction.

- Remind yourself that you are the boss, and that you will not allow a few strands of tobacco leaf to dominate and destroy your life.

- You must tell yourself repeatedly that you hate cigarettes and cultivate an aversion to smoking.

- You must develop an obsession with cigarette smoking cessation.

- Always remind yourself that you are "the master of tobacco and the captain of smoking."

Terminate Tobacco Tenaciously

Now that you have decided to quit smoking, there is no turning back. Set a date to exterminate cigarette smoking permanently and choose a timeframe for your emancipation from tobacco that is realistic and achievable. Give yourself a reasonable length of time to psych yourself up to stop smoking, for example, one to two weeks of a constant repetition of *"I hate cigarettes. I will not allow a stinky, dirty weed to rule me any longer. I am the master of my fate. I am the captain of my soul. Enough is enough."* You will develop an absolute hatred for cigarettes. You will have a complete aversion to tobacco.

Only YOU can stop your smoking. You can pay any amount of money to anybody you believe can help you stop your smoking, but the whole amount will be totally wasted because no-body can ever stop your smoking but you. Just like exercise, you have to do it yourself to gain the benefits. You will not derive any benefit from someone exercising on your behalf regardless of the sum of money you pay. You may gradually reduce or continue to smoke the same number of cigarettes over the one to two weeks that you are psyching yourself up to stop smoking completely.

I suspect most people will find it easier to gradually wean themselves off cigarettes. In the meantime, take advantage of this weaning period by saying to yourself, *"I hate cigarettes. I despise tobacco. I am determined to stop smoking by next Monday."* Write, *"I will stop smoking on* [the date you have chosen]*"* in big, bold, black capital letters on several white letter-sized pages and pin a copy in your office, bedroom, bathroom, dining room and living room. Repeatedly chant the date of your freedom from nicotine slavery to yourself. When the date of liberation from the evils of smoking arrives, you must be resolute. Stop smoking, period. No ifs, ands or butts—literally! You may chew gum, suck candies, bite toothpicks or your fingernails, whatever you must, but never, ever smoke again!

Congratulations! You've done it! You are now a proud reformed smoker. Within eight hours of the first day of your tobacco-free life, poisonous carbon monoxide disappears from your body and the oxygen level in your blood returns to normal. Within less than three days, you will be smelling roses and tasting cherries again. Your breathing will improve by at least 30% and your coughing will be reduced even more. In 10 years, the risk of dying from lung cancer will be reduced by 50%.[37] No less important is the psychological lift you get from the realization that you are the master of your fate and the captain of your soul.

My thoughts returned to Victor Patience and his wife. "You are absolutely correct to think that Victor probably wouldn't have had a stroke if he had stopped smoking even just a few hours earlier," I told Mrs. Patience.

She sniffed and dabbed at her eyes again. "Victor has always rationalized smoking by saying that he might suffer a stroke anyway because of the history of strokes in his family, including his father and an older brother. Do you believe that his genes conspired to cause his stroke?" Mrs. Patience now wondered.

Stop Smoking!

Acknowledge tobacco addiction
Commit to cigarette cessation
Terminate smoking tenaciously.

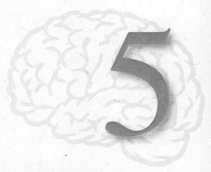

nurture over nature

"Nature can be modified by nurture;
even dogs can cease to relish meat
when they are trained to relish only vegetarian food."

~ Sri Sathya Sai Baba

"You cannot select your parents but you can elect their genes."

~ Felix Veloso

Prudence Patience said that her husband had always been afraid of suffering a stroke because of his genes. His father, paternal grandfather and several of his paternal uncles had had strokes. Mrs. Patience, a retired high school science teacher, knew the generally accepted modifiable risk factors for stroke—including hypertension, heart disease, diabetes, cigarette smoking, heavy alcohol consumption, high blood cholesterol levels and illicit drug abuse—that are correctable naturally without pharmaceuticals, and the customarily acknowledged unmodifiable risk factors for stroke, such as age, gender, race, heredity, and genetics.

The knowledgeable former school teacher further noted that

except for age, all the apparently unchangeable stroke risk factors are related to genetics. Mrs. Patience thought that her husband really needed not worry about his genetic predisposition to stroke since there was nothing he could have done to change his predicament.

"You don't worry about things you can't do anything about, right?" she observed philosophically. "Or is there something he could have done?" she wanted to know.

My mind reverted to the consultation I'd had with Gene Heritage about his fears regarding his genetic likelihood of stroke. Like Mrs. Patience, I'd met Mr. Heritage at the seminar I'd given a few weeks earlier. Gene Heritage was the retired insurance broker who'd needed a blood transfusion for internal bleeding caused by the aspirin he was taking to prevent stroke due to the strong history of brain attack in his family.

Like Mrs. Patience, Mr. Heritage had asked if there was anything he could do to remedy his supposedly unmodifiable risks for stroke, particularly the seemingly inflexible hereditary susceptibility to it. The anxious insurance agent was encouraged by information that new discoveries in the emerging sciences of *epigenetics* and *nutrigenomics* had revealed that innate traits can indeed be changed by environmental and dietary factors.[38]

Age is another risk factor that is perceived to be unchangeable. And it's true: the occurrence of stroke is directly proportional to age; the elderly are more likely to suffer a stroke. But it's *not* chronological age that is the main contributor to stroke incidence, it's biological or "virtual" age—the *real* age of the body that could be calculated as older or younger than chronological age depending on lifestyle and diet.

Gender is an unmodifiable risk factor, but the impact of the increased likelihood for males to suffer stroke can be mitigated by a healthy lifestyle and diet adjustments. Race and ethnicity probably play a role in stroke incidence—it is common knowledge that those of African descent have twice the rate of stroke compared to white North Americans,[39] but this difference may be partly accounted for by the fact that African Americans and Canadians are more prone to hypertension, diabetes mellitus and cigarette smoking—all of which are correctable stroke risk factors.

So, are conventional "unmodifiable" stroke risk factors, or even hereditary traits, potentially correctable? And if so, how?

While jogging on fallen leaves in Wascana Park one cold, cloudy autumn day, I gazed in amazement as flock after flock of Canada geese migrated south in V formation. It must be a vital instinct that drives them to hazard a winter flight of thousands of miles south where it is warm and food is plentiful. This same instinct for survival must compel them to also risk the return trip to their breeding ground in spring.

Loud and continuous honking drew my attention from the sky to the earth, where a few dozen Canada geese swam in the near-frozen water of Wascana lake. Why were these geese not instinctively taking wing to migrate to the south like their kin overhead? Surely, they too must notice the days getting shorter and the increasingly frigid temperatures that urged their cousins to find a warmer climate. After all, a wind chill of -40° Celsius must feel the same to a goose from up north as to a goose in Wascana Lake. So, why were the resident Wascana Canada geese staying in the cold? Part of the answer might be that the geese in Wascana Lake live the life of Riley: they're well fed both by the surrounding parkland and by human visitors, a few aerators in the man-made lake keep a small portion of the water unfrozen even in winter, and the park itself is a safe, protected environment. Northern geese *must* fly south to avoid starvation. The abundance of food around Wascana Lake has likely modified the genetic code of the Wascana geese so that they have lost their instinct to migrate. The new field of **nutrigenet-**

ics has proven that nutrition turns genes on or off, depending on the momentary needs of the creature.[40] The good life must have switched off the genes of their instinct to migrate.

Is there other evidence that genetic activity can be modified by environmental and nutritional factors?

I was jogging on a dirt farm road just outside of Wascana Park when two barking, snarling dogs charged menacingly toward me at a pace that seemed faster than thoroughbreds running in the Queen's Plate. I immediately came to a standstill, hoping that would turn off their chase instinct, but the huge dogs continued to barrel forward. Both canines (which turned out to be hunting dogs) were soon lunging for my throat. I had visions of my flesh being gnawed to shreds, but a loud command from their owner to "STOP!" silenced the growling brutes instantly. I was amazed. Why had the dogs obeyed? What halted their instinct to kill? The answer had to be training. But how does training switch off their genetic predatory instinct? Is heredity not inflexible? For a probable explanation, we have to ask to Pavlov.

Ivan Pavlov was a Russian physiologist who was awarded the 1904 Nobel Prize in medicine for his discoveries in the science of conditioned reflex. What Pavlov showed was that genetically determined reflexes can be modified by pairing a neutral trigger to the natural stimulus of a specific reflex. For example, the secretion of saliva is naturally triggered by the sight, smell, taste or mention of food but not by the ringing of a bell. Now, if a bell is rung consistently before each of a dog's meals, the canine will soon associate bell-ringing to feeding. In a short time, the dog salivates when the bell chimes and food is not needed to stimulate the salivary reflex anymore. The hereditary reflex of the secretion of digestive juices in response to the presence of food was modified to occur in response to a ringing sound. In other words, Pavlov altered the expression of the genes for digestion. And it was Pavlovian conditioning that stopped the hunting dogs from chewing me into ground meat. It is also Pavlovian conditioning that turns dogs from the predatory genes of their wolf cousins into the obedient behaviours that characterize man's best friend. How does Pavlovian conditioning change inherited genetic behaviour? The emerging science of epigenetics may provide the answer.

Epigenetics is the study of the processes that change the inheritable behaviour of a gene, especially its activation or deactivation, without directly affecting the makeup or DNA of the gene itself. Epigenetics has revealed the startling discovery that nutrients, toxins, behaviours and even the environment can modify our hereditary traits by silencing or activating the expression of our genes without altering our genetic code; the genetic structure remains unchanged but the physical, physiological and behavioral manifestations are modified.[41]

In embryonic development, signals to turn a gene on or off come from within the cell or between cells, but in later life environmental triggers such as diet, stress and physical activity (or lack thereof) play increasingly important roles. Epigeneticists are beginning to understand why genetically identical individuals develop different characteristics, such as a susceptibility to disease. Scientists have found that environmental exposure to nutritional, chemical and physical factors can alter the *epigenome*.

The classic comedy movie *Twins*, stars Arnold Schwarzenegger and Danny DeVito as twin brothers who grew up in completely different environmental, cultural, academic, physical, mental, dietary and financial situations and they developed to be totally opposite in appearance, behaviour, emotions, beliefs, reactions, psychology, ability, cognition and practices. That is epigenetics. Scientists are learning that healthy changes in lifestyle, nutrition, geographic location, environmental pollution and chemical exposure can modify an individual's innate risk factors for stroke. Several other chronic degenerative conditions, including obesity, heart disease, dementia and diabetes, are increasingly being recognized as epigenetic in nature. The migration of Canada geese and the obedience of the hunting dogs are evidence that environmental and experiential factors have modified the expression of these creatures' inherited genes.

But what about diet? Is there scientific evidence that diet can customize your heredity?

The nascent science of nutrigenomics says yes. **Nutrigenomics** examines both how the interaction between genetics and nutrition affects human health, and the influences of genes on the preferences for, and the metabolism and health consequences of, nutrition in humans. Nutrigenomicists see *nutrients* as codes that inform the cells of the body about the properties of the diet consumed. After the informed cells interpret the received nutritional data, they not only instruct certain genes to switch "on" or "off," but may even change their genome—their DNA— to conform to the situation, depending on the characteristics, quantity and quality of the nutrients in question, and the prevailing nutritional needs of the consumer. What is even more exciting is the possibility that dietary-induced genetic changes may be passed on to offspring.

I had explained all this to Mr. Heritage, who was amazed to learn that epigenetics and nutrigenomics could not only optimize genetic expressions, but may actually *improve* genetic structures. The retired insurance broker then wondered if there was any neurologic condition that might provide proof of the revolutionary epigenetic discovery that hereditary traits are modifiable by changes to lifestyle and diet. The treatment and effects of migraines immediately came to mind.

Migraine, an often familial headache syndrome with an up to 70% inheritance rate in some families, is characterized by recurrent attacks of usually severe, disabling, throbbing head pain frequently associated with nausea and vomiting, and a hypersensitivity to light, sound and smell. A migraine attack can be triggered by emotional, dietary, environmental or other factors. A study by Dr. Mikko Kallela of the Department of Neurology, Helsinki University Central Hospital found that identical twins with migraine experienced different headache characteristics that are not fully explained by genetic traits.[42] The most likely explanation for the differences in clinical symptoms of identical migraine genes is a disparity of environmental factors that epigenetics and nutrigenomics are continuing to unravel.

To better understand the influence of epigenetics and nutrigenomics on the manifestations of migraine in identical twins, let us review the upbringing of Nurture and her twin sister, Nature, whose biological parents are both migraine sufferers. The girls were separated shortly after birth. Nurture was adopted by a wealthy, happily married couple, both of whom suffered frequent debilitating migraine attacks and therefore learned to avoid common migraine triggers, including: cheese; alcohol— especially red wine; chocolate; processed meats such as hot dogs; irregular sleep patterns; hunger; fragrances; bright, glaring lights; fatigue; and psychological stress.

Nature, however, grew up in a migraine-free environment. She was fostered by emotionally stretched and financially strained hard-working parents who nevertheless did not suffer headaches and were therefore ignorant of migraine and its triggers. Nature grew up eating and drinking whatever and whenever she liked. She was also free to sleep for as long or as short as her busy schedule permitted.

Now, imagine these identical twins comparing notes on their migraine frequency, severity, duration and responsiveness to treatment when they met for the first time to celebrate their twentieth birthdays. I'll give you only one guess as to which of the identical twins suffers the least from migraines.

If you voted for Nurture over Nature, you are now secure in the knowledge that even though you cannot choose your parents, you can select the expression of their genes by living and eating healthily.

The conclusion that heredity is not the absolute determinant of your fate is further supported by the New England centenarian study of 1,600 people who have lived 100 years or more, which found that "150 longevity genes" and healthy lifestyles—including regular exercise, good diet and avoidance of tobacco—are responsible for life longevity. The research confirmed that healthy lifestyles are critical to a long and healthy life, regardless of the particular genetic advantages a person might have.[43]

Perhaps even Charles Darwin's *Origin of the Species,* based on the survival of the fittest via natural selection, evolved through epigenetics and nutrigenomics.

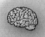

Nurture Yourself

You cannot select your parents but you can elect their genes by healthy living and eating.

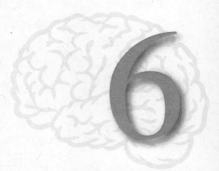

healthercise

*"Lack of activity destroys the good condition
of every human being, while movement and
methodical physical exercise save it and preserve it."*

~ PLATO

*"Those who think they have not time for bodily exercise
will sooner or later have to find time for illness."*

~ EDWARD STANLEY

Based on Prudence Patience's information, I was now sure
that her husband's stroke had occurred exactly one-and-a-half
hours earlier. We had only 90 minutes left to complete our assessment and safely administer tPA to Mr. Patience. But we still
needed his consent to give him the life-saving treatment. And
he had asked the stroke nurse to contact his son for the consent.

"Mrs. Patience, do you have your son's telephone number?"
I asked, "I have to contact him right away to get his consent to
treat your husband with tPA."

"Yes," she nodded, opening her purse and pulling out a little
black book, "I always carry my address book and important

phone numbers with me. Here's my son's number," she said, handing over the book. I took it with me to the phone at the emergency admitting desk and waited for the call to be picked up. It was Saturday and I hoped their son was home.

"Dr. Patrick Patience's residence," a female voice answered. I remembered then that Mrs. Patience had told me her son was a doctor of pharmacy.

"Hello. This is Dr. Felix Veloso calling from Regina. There's an emergency—Dr. Patience's father just had a stroke. I must speak to him right away to get consent to treat his father."

"Oh no!" said the woman, who explained she was Dr. Patience's wife. "Patrick's not here! He's gone for a run on the seawall around Stanley Park," she added.

"Does he have a cell phone with him?" I asked urgently.

"Yes. Here's the number," she said, reciting the digits.

As I dialed the long-distance number, my mind flashed back 30 years earlier to another morning jog interrupted by an emergency. There were no cell phones in those days and the message on my pager had requested I call the hospital immediately. I'd rushed to the emergency room instead since I was nowhere near a telephone.

The head nurse met me at the door and breathlessly informed me that the only grandson of a well-known politician had just had a stroke. I immediately proceeded to examine the 18-year-old patient, not taking time to acknowledge the presence of the distinguished gentleman standing by the bedside until he asked, "Are you the neurologist?" I instantly recognized him as the most prominent cabinet minister of the provincial government of the day. Outfitted in T-shirt, running shoes and shorts and sweating profusely from the heat of the sunny, summer day, I was a far cry from the Hollywood image of a physician. No wonder he wanted to confirm my identity!

"Yes," I said, apologizing and introducing myself to the politician. "Sorry to rush here in my jogging gear."

"You must be an avid ParticipACTIONer," he surmised, taking in the worn state of my runners, "in which case I thank you for setting an example for your patients and colleagues both."

This surprised me; I had been prepared for a brusque comment about professional attire but was thrilled to be congratulated instead. I subsequently learned that this cabinet minister was not only a strong supporter of ParticipACTION but had also vigorously promoted Saskatoon, Saskatchewan as ParticipACTION's first model community to assess the extent of possible cooperation of local public and private sectors in a fitness program.[a]

Investigation revealed that the politician's grandson had a hole in the wall of his heart that separated the right side from the left. This congenital condition, *patent foramen ovale,* allows blood clots in the right half of the heart, which should normally go to the lungs, to detour to the left side of the heart and from there to the brain, causing stroke. The hole in the teenager's heart was subsequently closed by our excellent team of heart surgeons and the patient had recovered nicely from the stroke without any significant disability.

Now, as I waited impatiently for Patrick Patience to answer his cell phone, I asked his mother, "Does Victor exercise?"

She nodded. "Victor joined ParticipACTION at the same time Patrick did but just didn't have the determination to exercise regularly," she lamented. "It's the same as his smoking—Victor doesn't have the willpower to persevere. Oh, he enrolled in lots of fitness classes and attended several exercise programs, but he'd always quit after a few weeks, disappointed at not having lost any weight despite his efforts. I've explained to him time and again that exercise takes a while to work, but he is easily discouraged. He also has plenty of excuses too.

a The project ran for six years from 1972 to 1978 and was tremendously successful in showing that locally generated funds and volunteers can sustain a community fitness program. The Saskatoon ParticipACTION model was later copied by communities across Canada and around the world.

"'No time,' he says. Can you imagine? He's retired and says he has no time to exercise! Reminds me of a poster that reads: 'Those who do not have time for exercise will have to make time for sickness.' He also claims we can't afford the cost of sports equipment or gym memberships, yet his cigarettes cost at least $10 a day! Oh! And he also claims there's no place for him to exercise safely, especially in poor weather. But our son set up a state-of-the-art gym for him, including an excellent foldable treadmill that measures heart rate, speed, distance, calories burned, time run, etc. It even has a TV in the console," she concluded.

I could hear the worry warring with exasperation in her voice. Victor Patience was a man who had had every opportunity to exercise and reduce his risk factors for stroke, yet he hadn't taken advantage of them.

"TURN-OFF YOUR CELL PHONE," said the poster by the entrance to the hospital auditorium where I presided over a question-and-answer session for the Hospital's Women Auxiliary titled "Fitness is Your Responsibility, No One Else's."

I had opened the meeting by telling the audience about an athletic middle-aged lady who stopped her run to speak to a grandfatherly-looking man cheerfully wishing passing joggers a nice day. "Excuse me, sir, I can't help noticing how happy you are. What's your secret for a long and happy life?"

"I smoke two packs of cigarettes every day," the elderly man replied. "I also drink 24 ounces of whisky and eat three high calorie, fatty meals a day. But I pay $1,000 a month to a personal trainer to do my daily exercise," the aged man boasted.

"That's incredible," the jogger said. "How old are you?"

"Almost twenty-five!" the old man proudly proclaimed.

There was polite laughter. I had been pleased that the audience realized that exercise is a serious endeavour and that the benefits of fitness accumulate only for the exerciser and no one else. The attendees also recognized that:

- life is motion
- all living things move
- the force for movement must come from within the self
- all living creatures are constantly in motion
- to be alive means to be active
- activities cease when life stops
- death is motionless.

I quoted Zun Xi, a Chinese philosopher from the 3rd century B.C.: "If you take good care of yourself and exercise regularly, heaven cannot make you ill. If you do not do so, heaven cannot make you healthy."

A retired social worker stood up and told the audience that her husband, who had all the major risk factors for stroke except for smoking—he'd quit after a heart attack two years earlier—paid for expensive drugs (all with serious side effects) for high blood pressure, diabetes, weight reduction and high cholesterol, but could not exercise because of unstable angina.[b] Despite all the medications, he had recently had a warning stroke. The distraught lady went on to say that her husband would undoubtedly be willing to pay a surrogate dearly if only the health benefits of exercise were transferable.

BENEFITS OF REGULAR EXERCISE

- helps prevent heart disease
- lowers the risk of developing diabetes mellitus
- improves blood sugar control for diabetics
- normalizes blood pressure

---

b A heart condition marked by paroxysms of chest pain due to reduced oxygen to the heart.

- lessens the risk of developing cancer, particularly cancer of the breast, prostate and colon
- aids in successful weight control
- provides stress relief
- helps prevent osteoporosis
- elevates *high-density lipoprotein (HDL)* levels (good cholesterol)
- reduces *low-density lipoprotein (LDL)* levels (bad cholesterol)
- prevents falls in elderly adults by promoting muscle strength, flexibility, agility and balance.
- enhances psychological and emotional well-being
- promotes restorative, restful sleep
- improves memory
- delays development of dementia
- is 20% better than angioplasty[c] in stable coronary artery disease patients.[44]

After I listed the benefits, she wanted to know if there was any proof that exercise can prevent stroke.

"Absolutely," I replied. "Numerous studies have shown regular exercise reduces the occurrence of stroke."

Regular Exercise Reduces the Occurence of Stroke

- A Honolulu Heart Program study of 8,006 middle-aged and elderly men found regular exercise protects against stroke.[45]

- A Physicians' Health Study of 21, 823 men followed for 11.1 years found vigorous exercise is associated with a decreased stroke risk in men.[46]

---

c An operation in which a blocked artery is opened with a balloon.

- The Nurses' Health Study of 72,488 female nurses in 11 U.S. states reported that even just moderate-intensity exercise such as walking is associated with a substantial reduction of stroke risk.[47]

- A meta-analysis of 23 studies of physical activities and stroke risks by Dr. Chong Do Lee and his colleagues from the Department of Sport and Exercise Sciences of West Texas A&M University revealed that active individuals lower their stroke risk by at least 25% compared to their more sedentary cohorts.[48]

- The Northern Manhattan Stroke Study by Dr. Ralph Sacco and his colleagues from Columbia University College of Physicians and Surgeons in New York found that moderate intensity physical activity reduces the occurrence of stroke in elderly individuals regardless of gender or ethnicity.[49]

- A sub-analysis of the Framingham Study demonstrated that moderate intensity physical activity reduces the relative risks of stroke occurrence by 41%.[50]

- The National Health and Nutrition Examination Survey I (NHANES I) Epidemiologic Follow-up Study, of 7,895 white people and black people aged 45–74 years, conducted by Dr. Richard Gillum and associates from the National Center for Health Statistics, Centers for Disease Control and Prevention, found that regular physical activity prevents stroke in men and women regardless of colour.[51]

- A study by Dr. E. Lindenstrom and associates from the Department of Neurology of Rigshospital in Copenhagen, Denmark titled "Lifestyle factors and risk of cerebrovascular disease in women. The Copenhagen City Heart Study" showed that lack of exercise increases the relative risk of stroke to 1.4, which is alarmingly similar to that of cigarette smoking.[52]

- Dr. J. Z. Willey and associates from Columbia University in New York and the Miller School of Medicine in Miami in a report titled "Physical activity and risk of ischemic stroke in the Northern Manhattan Study" reported that older individuals, especially males, performing 20 to 40 minutes of moderate intensity physical activity three to five days a week are 63% less likely to suffer a stroke compared to people who do no physical activity. The Northern Manhattan Study is a prospective cohort study of 3,298 older, urban-dwelling, multi-ethnic, stroke-free individuals followed for 9.1 years.[53]

- Another study by Jacob Sattelmair and colleagues at Harvard School of Public Health in Boston of more than 39,000 healthy women aged 45 or older enrolled in the Women's Health Study for 12 years found that active women who walked two or more hours a week at any pace cut their risk of any type of stroke by 30%, and women who walked at a pace of three miles per hour or faster benefited even more, with an additional 37% lower risk of suffering any type of stroke compared to those who walked at a slower pace.[54]

Exercise Fosters New Brain Cell Growth

More importantly—and contrary to the belief that injury to the approximately 100 billion brain cells from whatever cause is permanent and dead nerve cells are not replaced by new ones—recent studies have shown that **regular exercise fosters new brain cell growth and promotes repair of damaged nerve cells** by stimulating the release of a nerve growth factor called *brain-derived neurotrophic factor* (BDNF), a major neurotrophin that supports the repair, growth, function and survival of neurons. Regular exercise also reduces the levels of harmful *myelin-associated glycoprotein* (MAG) and *Nogo-A*, proteins specific to the brain which inhibit the growth of new nerve fibres needed to connect nerve cells, allowing for the free flow of electrical messages between them.[55]

Fernando Gómez-Pinilla and co-investigators from the Department of Physiological Science, Division of Neurosurgery, UCLA Brain Injury Research Center and Brain Research Institute, Los Angeles, California reported that exercise in mice can promote changes in *neuroplasticity*—also known as cortical remapping, the ability of the human brain to change based on experience—via increased levels of BDNF. Dr. Gómez-Pinilla also found that exercise may help reverse some of the damage of traumatic brain injury in rodents by reducing the levels of proteins that inhibit new neural growth and by increasing levels of the protein that enhances such growth.[56]

Dr. Muriel Koehl of the French National Institute for Health and Medical Research at the University of Bordeaux and colleagues at Northwestern University and the University of Groningen in Haren, the Netherlands, found that *beta-endorphin*—a mood-elevating chemical produced by the *hypothalamus* and the *pituitary gland*—released during exercise may be a key factor in promoting the exertion's nerve cell growth-stimulating effect on the brain. Dr. Koehl also found that exercise creates new neurons in the *hippocampus*, a brain region involved in learning and memory which may explain the increased learning and memory, performances observed in people who exercise.[57]

Dr. Michael Davis at the University of Texas Health Science Center showed that regular exercise provided an approximately 35% improvement in brain blood flow after a stroke in rats.[58]

The theory is that exercise promotes new blood vessel growth, which increases cerebral blood flow, which, in turn, helps protect against damage from ischemic stroke.

There is solid evidence proving that exercise not only prevents nerve cell damage caused by stroke but may also repair it. There is currently no drug available that both prevents and treats stroke, which is the first cause of permanent disability[59] and the second highest cause of death.[60]

Studies have also confirmed that exercise not only prevents but may be better than angioplasty for those with *coronary heart disease*, which is the leading cause of death in Canada.[61] Researchers also found that exercise prevents cancer,[62] which is the third highest cause of mortality.[63]

"Indeed," I told the audience, "exercise appears to be the fountain of youth that Ponce de Leon searched for far and wide but could not find. All he needed to do was simply make use of his arms and legs!"

Another hand went up. "Dr. Veloso, I was recently diagnosed with prehypertension. My family doctor recommended that I start an exercise program and also reduce salt intake to prevent the progression of my borderline high blood pressure. He also said that since—like 65% of adults in North America[64]—I have been living a sedentary lifestyle, I should start with moderate intensity exercise before progressing to more strenuous workouts. But I don't know what moderate or vigorous exercises are. Could you please define light, moderate and vigorous activities?" asked a retired medical records librarian.

Her predicament was echoed by several others in the audience. Most exercise and weight reduction programs almost always advise starting with light exercise before progressing to moderate then high intensity activities but usually never describe the intensity of the workout.

"All you need to remember is that **light exercises** are activities that do not cause any breathlessness and burn 50 to 200 calories per hour.[d] Taking a leisurely walk around the neighbourhood is a prime example of light exercise. If you dance, then doing the rhumba or a slow waltz would be excellent choices for light exercise. Another superb—and productive!—light exercise is housecleaning."

There was a ripple of laughter and a few groans from the crowd.

I went on. "**Moderate exercises** use 200 to 350 calories per hour. A brisk walk around the park that leaves you slightly breathless but able to converse comfortably is moderate exercise. If you are a dancer, the cha-cha is a fabulous moderate intensity exercise. Other example of moderate exercises are swimming, biking, bowling, canoeing, gardening and golfing—if you pull your own cart.

"**Vigorous exercises** require an exertion of over 350 calories per hour. Participating in a walk-a-thon or dancing the jive are activities that easily qualify as strenuous exercises. Others are badminton, singles tennis, jogging, squash, skating and skiing."

"But what is the *best* exercise?" the same lady wanted to know.

When I started my own fitness plan 40 years earlier I'd been

---

d There are two forms of calories, both of which are units of heat energy. The "small" or "gram" calorie—the amount of energy needed to heat one gram of water by one degree Celsius—is used often in science, but is too small to conveniently describe the energy content of food, so the "kilocalorie" is used instead and is, confusingly, called simply a Calorie in dietary terminology.

The "food" calorie equals 1000 "gram" calories. The food or "kilogram" calorie represents the amount of energy needed to raise the temperature of a kilogram of water by one degree. Any mention of "calorie" in this book refers to the larger "food" calorie. See also: http://en.wikipedia.org/wiki/calorie. Accessed October 17, 2010.

told that jogging was probably the best exercise, except if you were a fish, in which case swimming was definitely healthier. Today my answer is that everybody is different and that the best exercise for anyone is one that is customized, individualized and personalized to that unique person's current physical, psychological and environmental circumstances.

"Whatever activity you find most enjoyable, practicable and doable at the time is the 'best' exercise for you," I told her.

"Is there a minimum amount of exercise that must be completed to be beneficial?" the retired librarian wanted to clarify.

I thought about it. "If we agree that exercise is any physical exertion over and above your customary activities of daily living, then any exercise—be it light, moderate or intense and of any duration—is healthy. However, most experts advise at least 30 minutes of moderate intensity exercise three times a week for optimal health benefits," I said.

"So, Dr. Veloso, if even minimal exercise is healthy, can you exercise too much?" she then asked.

"Yes," I replied and then reminded the audience of Paracelsus, the respected Renaissance physician who cautioned that "too much of anything will hurt you," and of Roman playwright Terence's teaching of "moderation in all things."

"Listen to your body—it will guide you to your optimum degree of exercise," I said. In general:

- exercises that are uncomfortable should be avoided
- the intensity level of painful physical activities ought to be reduced
- the duration of exhausting activities must be shortened to reserve vital resources so permanent bodily damage does not occur.

"What about marathons?" she went on. "Don't some apparently healthy runners suddenly die of heart attack during marathons? Isn't this a warning against strenuous aerobic exercise?"

"While it is true that rare deaths have occurred during marathon events, the fatalities are few and far between, and the benefits from running the race far outweigh the risk of fatality.

"In fact, a study published in the *British Medical Journal* by Dr. Donald Redelmeier, a professor of medicine at the University of Toronto, found that in 26 randomly selected established North American marathons from 1975 to 2004 and including about 3.3 million runners, there were only 26 deaths. That's an average of 0.8 fatalities per 100,000 marathoners," I said.

"The victims were typically middle-aged males who usually died near the end of the race and almost all were subsequently discovered to have been suffering from hardening of the arteries. The researchers further placed the data in perspective by stating that approximately two deaths occur for every million hours of aerobic exercise, compared to around 20 motor vehicle fatalities for every million hours of driving. The study clearly shows that aerobic exercise is healthier and safer than driving,"[65] I explained.

The retired librarian then commented that she had always been told that exercise was meant to keep her physically fit. "Fit for what?" she wanted to know.

I chuckled, as did several others, but did my best to answer. "Depending on the context, *physical fitness* usually means a state of healthy well-being that allows an individual to live a good quality of life. Physical fitness is the vitality to live. Physical fitness may also refer to specific fitness levels—the capability to perform a particular task, such as driving. In short, specific fitness is the ability to work," I said.

An athletic-looking lady in her late fifties spoke up. "We are enthusiastic practitioners of ParticipACTION to stay healthy. My husband and I exercise at least 30 minutes three times a week, as recommended by the experts. But I find I often have difficulty falling asleep, especially after a workout late in the day. We've gone to many fitness classes and are always encouraged to keep physically active, but we never hear a word about rest and sleep. Isn't it also important for our health to rest and to sleep regularly?" she asked.

I nodded. "Just as our bodies need activity to stay healthy, we also require regular rest periods and adequate sleep. We often forget that our bodies need rest to restore energy and maintain vitality. We also need sufficient sleep to keep our minds and bodies working at maximum efficiency. Taking a 20- to 30-minute 'siesta' after lunch is a great way to refresh your vigour and alertness. For most adults, the optimum number of hours of sleep is between seven to nine hours. Dim your bedroom lights about half an hour before going to bed to allow your brain to increase the production of *melatonin*. **Melatonin** is a natural hormone secreted mostly by the tiny pineal gland located in the centre of the brain. Melatonin is not only a powerful hypnotic but is also a strong antioxidant, antidepressant and immunomodulator.[e] Light inhibits and darkness stimulates melatonin production. If dimming your bedroom light is not enough to help you fall asleep easily, then you might want to try commercially available melatonin. The standard dose of melatonin to induce sleep is 3 mg. taken about 15 to 30 minutes before going to bed.[f] Needless to say, you should avoid exercising late in the day," I responded.

"Please excuse my ignorance, but what is ParticipACTION?" asked a petite woman.

"It's a bit of a long story," I said. "To better understand ParticipACTION's roots, we need to have a basic history of Canada's universal health care system. For a variety of reasons, including its notoriously long, cold winter, Saskatchewan has had a history of a shortage of doctors to staff its equally scarce hospitals.

e A natural or synthetic substance that helps regulate or normalize the immune system.

f Melatonin may cause drowsiness so you must not take it prior to activities that require alertness, such as driving. Melatonin may react with some medications. Consult your doctor before taking melatonin.

In 1946, the Co-operative Commonwealth Federation (CCF) government, under the leadership of Tommy Douglas, passed the *Saskatchewan Hospitalization Act*, which guaranteed free hospital care for much of the population.

"Saskatchewan was, until recently, a 'have-not' province and could not afford the universal health care that the CCF government had hoped to provide. In 1957, the federal government passed the *Hospital Insurance and Diagnostic Services Act* to fund 50% of the cost of any provincial government health care program. The premier of Saskatchewan at the time, Mr. Woodrow Lloyd, decided to use this federal grant to fund the long-aspired-to universal health program to include coverage for both physicians' fees and hospitalization costs. Saskatchewan's pioneering universal health care program proved to be a great success and was soon demanded by other provinces. The Liberal federal government under Lester B. Pearson, then prime minister, introduced the *Medical Care Act* in 1966, which expanded the *Hospital Insurance and Diagnostic Services Act*'s cost-sharing, allowing provinces to establish universal health care plans.[66]

"In 1984, parliament passed the *Canada Health Act,* which mandates that the provincial universal health care plan must be comprehensive, universal, portable, accessible and publicly administered, and prohibits user fees as well as extra billing by doctors. In 1975, 10 years after the establishment of the universal health care plan, the total Canadian health care cost was 7% of the Gross Domestic Product (GDP). Thirty years later, in 2005, Canada's total health care grew to an estimated 10.4% of GDP or the equivalent of about $4,411 CDN per person. In 1975, 45% of the total health care cost was consumed by hospitals, 15% was paid to physicians and 9% was spent on pharmaceuticals. Three decades later, in 2005, hospital charges declined from 45 to 30%, physicians' costs were reduced from 15 to 13%, but the cost of pharmaceuticals doubled from 9% to 18% of total Canadian health care expenditures.[67]

"Alarmed by Canada's widespread and increasingly sedentary lifestyle and the growing obesity epidemic that in 2001 added an estimated cost of $5.3 billion to the total expenditure of Canada's universal health program, in 1972, Prime Minister Pierre Trudeau launched ParticipACTION. Its mandate was to promote healthy living and physical fitness. After 30 years of remarkable success in transforming unfit and inactive Canadians like myself into a nation of physical fitness enthusiasts, the program was suspended because of lack of funding. Thankfully—and healthfully!—ParticipACTION was re-instituted in February 2007 after Ontario Health said that 50% of adults in that province were overweight, and that the direct and indirect costs of treating obesity-related chronic health problems—particularly diabetes mellitus and its complications—amounted to $1.6 billion annually.[68]

Another hand went up. "Doctor, you said there was no 'best' exercise, but is there a 'perfect' exercise?" asked a plump lady in her mid-sixties.

I smiled. "I am not an exercise expert but I *would* be pleased to share with you my opinion that *Tai Chi Chuan*, the ancient Chinese system of gentle movement patterns, is the perfect exercise. I believe that Tai Chi Chuan, which I prefer to translate as 'Supreme Ultimate Healthercise' instead of the literal translation of 'Supreme Ultimate Force,' can minimize the looming health care crisis of our rapidly aging population, who will inevitably be afflicted with degenerative illnesses needing expensive long-term care."

The idea of "supreme ultimate" is associated with the Chinese concept of yin/yang, the belief that opposites create one another and are mutually dependent. *Tai Chi Chuan* may be viewed as the tangible art form of the dynamic duality of *yin* and *yang* (male/female, active/passive, dark/light, forceful/yielding, hard/

soft) in everything. **Tai Chi Chuan** borrows the yin/yang circle of life symbol as its own icon.

The Tai Chi Chuan symbol means that everything in the universe (the "Ten Thousand Things" of the *Tao Te Ching* by Lao Tzu) contains both light and dark, good and evil. These are complementary aspects rather than conflicting ones. The two small dots within each area indicate that yin contains the seed of yang, and yang contains the seed of yin.

"Force" here is translated to *chi*, which, in Traditional Chinese Medicine (TCM), is the vital force that animates the body. This "chi" circulates in patterns that are closely related to the nervous and vascular systems, and thus the approach is closely connected with acupuncture. Health in TCM depends on a correct balance of yin/yang and a proper flow of chi around the body. Illness and death result from a lack or blockage of chi flow in the body. Tai Chi Chuan, with its mental discipline and precise execution of postural exercises, promises spiritual and physical benefits by channeling this vital energy.

You need not subscribe to the Chinese yin/yang and chi beliefs to benefit from exercising Tai Chi Chuan. Practising Tai Chi Chuan provides an easy, safe, effective and inexpensive avenue for improving balance, alignment, motor control, rhythm of movement, flexibility, mobility and range of motion. There is evidence that indicates that Tai Chi Chuan enriches cardiovascular endurance, improves posture, reinforces strength and enhances balance. Numerous scientific studies show that it has the same healthy benefits as brisk walking on heart rate, blood pressure and circulation.[69] Tai Chi Chuan has been called "meditation in motion."[70] The calming, relaxing, meditative nature of the Tai Chi Chuan exercise promotes the *relaxation response,* the exact opposite of the *fight* or *flight response* provoked by stress. Tai Chi Chuan is therefore a potent stress reliever.

Tai Chi Chuan can be practised in the comfort of your home during inclement weather or, preferably, in the wide open space of a park where you may also enjoy the soothing sights, sounds, and smells of nature, breathe fresh clean air and bathe in bright sunlight. It may be performed in peaceful solitude or enjoyed in tranquility with friends. Many movements in the Tai Chi Chuan repertoire can be performed lying down, sitting or standing. The gentleness of Tai Chi Chuan allows even the severely disabled to adapt at least a few forms of the exercise to their routine. Several Tai Chi Chuan patterns, particularly the breathing exercises, can be enjoyed anywhere and any time, including at work, during coffee or lunch breaks, while seated on buses, riding in trains or traveling in airplanes. Although preferably performed early in the morning, Tai Chi Chuan may be enjoyed any time of the day that you are not busy. It does not require expensive, special outfits or equipment. Tai Chi Chuan is the ultimate body and mind tonic. Truly, as devotees of the art know, Tai Chi Chuan is the Supreme Ultimate Healthercise.

The history of Tai Chi Chuan has been obscured by antiquity. There are many conflicting stories about its origins, but the most romantic version is that it was created by a Taoist monk named Chang San-feng about 700 years ago.

It is said that Chang San-feng wanted to develop a system of exercise that would strengthen the body and enlighten the minds of Buddhist monks who were physically weakened by spending most of their waking hours in sedentary prayer and were therefore defenseless against the numerous marauding bandits roaming the countryside where the majority of monasteries were located.

One story tells how he dreamed of a combat between a snake and a crane. In life, the snake would be easy prey for the crane. In his dream, Chang was greatly impressed by the retreating/advancing and the yielding/evading tactics employed by the snake to escape the attack of the crane, then striking when the crane was in its most vulnerable stance. In Chang's dream, when the crane attacked the snake's head, the snake evaded it and hit the bird with its tail. When the crane tried for the snake's tail, the snake bit the crane.

The retreating and advancing manoeuvres employed by the snake reminded Chang of China's most fundamental philosophy of yin and yang, the concept that opposites create one another and are mutually dependent. The dream inspired Chang San-feng to develop the basic Tai Chi Chuan's concepts of evading, yielding, sticking and attacking, and he created a martial art that used softness and internal power to overcome brute force. Chang jealously guarded his creation and taught his martial art only to members of his clan.

Yang Lu-Chan (1799 - 1872) wanted desperately to learn Tai Chi Chuan but Chang San-feng only taught members of his family. So Yang took a job as a servant in the Chang household and learned Tai Chi by surreptitiously watching the Changs performed the patterns at night. Later, alone in his room, he practised what he had observed. One day he was discovered and asked to show what he had secretly learned. The Changs were greatly impressed by Yang's Tai Chi performance and decided to formally teach him the complete routine.

Historians say that Yang studied Tai Chi under the Changs for at least six and perhaps up to 18 years. Yang then returned to his hometown of Kuang Ping where he taught Chang San-feng's style of Tai Chi to others. His fame as a Tai Chi master soon attracted the attention of the emperor, who invited Yang to be the military martial arts teacher for the Manchu government. The original Chang San-feng's Tai Chi style consisted of 13 postures, based on the eight *trigrams*, or philosophical concepts, of the *I Ching* or *Book of Changes* and Feng Shui's five elements of Wood, Fire, Earth, Metal and Water. This proved to be too rough-and-tumble for the imperial court so Yang modified the movements to a more gentle, graceful routine of exercises known as Yang's Style Long Form, consisting of 103 postures and taking about 20 minutes to perform.[71]

The 103 postures of Yang-style Tai Chi Chuan	
1.	Preparation Form
2.	Beginning
3.	Grasp the Bird's Tail
4.	Single Whip
5.	Lift Hands and Step Up
6.	White Crane Spreads Its Wings
7.	Brush Knee, Left
8.	Hand Plays Pipa
9.	Brush Knee, Left
10.	Brush Knee, Right
11.	Brush Knee, Left
12.	Play Pipa
13.	Brush Knee, Left
14.	Step Forward, Deflect, Parry and Punch (as though) Sealed and Closed
15.	Appears Closed (Rufeng Sibi), Withdraw and Push as if Closing a Door
16.	Cross Hands
17.	Embrace Tiger and Return to Mountain
18.	Fist Under Elbow
19.	Repulse Monkey, Left
20.	Repulse Monkey, Right
21.	Repulse Monkey, Left
22.	Diagonal Flying
23.	Lift Hands and Step Up
24.	White Crane Lifts Wings
25.	Brush Knee, Left and Step
26.	Pick up Needle from Bottom of Sea
27.	Fan Penetrates Back
28.	Turn Body and Flip Fist Past Body
29.	Step Forward, Deflect, Parry and Punch
30.	Step Up and Grasp the Bird's Tail
31.	Single Whip

32.	Wave Hands like Cloud, Left
33.	Wave Hands like Cloud, Right
34.	Wave Hands like Cloud, Left
35.	Single Whip
36.	High Pat on Horse
37.	Right Separate Foot
38.	Left Separate Foot
39.	Turn Body, Left Heel Kick
40.	Brush Knee, Left and Step
41.	Brush Knee, Right and Step
42.	Step Up and Punch Down
43.	Turn Body and Flip Fist Past Body
44.	Step Forward, Deflect, Parry and Punch
45.	Right Heel Kick
46.	Strike Tiger, Left
47.	Strike Tiger, Right
48.	Turn Body, Right Heel Kick
49.	Strike to Ears with Both Fists
50.	Left Heel Kick
51.	Turn Body, Right Heel Kick
52.	Step Forward, Deflect, Parry and Punch (as though) Sealed and Closed
53.	Appears Closed (Rufeng Sibi), Withdraw and Push as if Closing a Door
54.	Cross Hands
55.	Embrace Tiger and Return to Mountain
56.	Diagonal Single Whip
57.	Part the Wild Horse's Mane, Right
58.	Part the Wild Horse's Mane, Left
59.	Part the Wild Horse's Mane, Right
60.	Grasp the Bird's Tail
61.	Single Whip
62.	Jade Lady Passes Through the Shuttle
63.	Grasp the Bird's Tail
64.	Single Whip
65.	Wave Hands like Cloud, Left
66.	Wave Hands like Cloud, Right
67.	Wave Hands like Cloud, Left
68.	Single Whip
69.	Snake Creeps Down

70.	Golden Rooster Stands On One Leg, Left
71.	Golden Rooster Stands On One Leg, Right
72.	Repulse Monkey, Left
73.	Repulse Monkey, Right
74.	Repulse Monkey, Left
75.	Diagonal Flying
76.	Lift Hands and Step Up
77.	White Crane Lifts Wings
78.	Left Brush Knee and Step
79.	Pick up Needle from Bottom of Sea
80.	Fan Penetrates Back
81.	Turn Body, White Snake Spits Tongue
82.	Step Forward, Deflect, Parry and Punch
83.	Step Up and Grasp the Bird's Tail
84.	Single Whip
85.	Wave Hands like Cloud, Left
86.	Wave Hands like Cloud, Right
87.	Wave Hands like Cloud, Left
88.	Single Whip
89.	High Pat on Horse with Palm Thrust
90.	Cross Kick
91.	Step Forward and Punch Groin
92.	Step Up and Grasp the Bird's Tail
93.	Single Whip
94.	Snake Creeps Down
95.	Step Up to Seven Stars
96.	Step Back and Ride Tiger
97.	Turn Body and Swing Over Lotus
98.	Bend Bow and Shoot Tiger
99.	Step Forward, Deflect, Parry and Punch (as though) Sealed and Closed
100.	Appears Closed (Rufeng Sibi), Withdraw and Push as if Closing a Door
101.	Cross Hands
102.	Closing (Shoushi)
103.	Return to Normal

It is generally accepted that the North Americanization of Tai Chi Chuan was led by Cheng Man-Ching, commonly regarded as the most brilliant student of the Yang-style Long Form.

Cheng Man-Ching taught in New York where he wrote several books on Tai Chi, including the famous *Cheng's 13 Chapters on Tai-Chi Chuan*. Cheng Man-Ching modified Yang-style Long Form from 103 to 37 postures by eliminating repetition so as to shorten the time to complete the routine to approximately 10 minutes while enhancing the health benefits of the exercise.[72]

The 37 postures of Cheng Man-Ching's Tai Chi Style
1.   Preparation: stand straight with eyes looking ahead and feet slightly apart
2.   Beginning: raise hands back and down
3.   Ward Off, Left
4.   Ward Off, Right
5.   Roll Back: a defensive posture useful for the small to overcome the big
6.   Press: to transmit power through the wrist of the other hand
7.   Push: the knee and elbow coordinate in this manoeuvre. Postures 3 through 7 are collectively known as "grasping bird's tail," which gives the impression of a person inspecting a bird
8.   Single Whip: a posture promoting chi circulation
9.   Raise Hands
10. Shoulder Stroke: great close-contact fighting technique
11. White Crane Spreads Wings
12. Brush Knee, Left
13. Play Pipa. Repeat Brush Knee, Left
14. Step Up and Block
15. Parry and Punch
16. Withdraw and Push
17. Cross Hands
18. Embrace Tiger, Return to Mountain. Roll Back, Press, Push, then Single Whip in the direction of the corner (diagonal)
19. Fist Under Elbow
20. Step Back and Repulse Monkey, Right
21. Step Back and Repulse Monkey, Left. Repulse Monkey, Right. Repulse Monkey, Left. Repulse Monkey, Right
22. Diagonal Flying
23. Wave Hands Like Clouds, Right

24. Wave Hands Like Clouds, Left. Wave Hands Like Clouds, Right Wave Hands Like Clouds, Left
25. Snake Creeps Down
26. Golden Rooster Stands on One Leg, Right
27. Golden Rooster Stands on One Leg, Left
28. Separation of the Right Foot
29. Separation of the Left Foot
30. Turn Body and Kick With Heel. Brush Knee, Left. Brush Knee, Right
31. Step Forward and Punch. Step up into Ward Off, Right. Roll Back, Press, Push and Single Whip
32. Fair Lady Weaves Shuttle I
33. Fair Lady Weaves Shuttle II These postures are followed by Fair Lady Weaves Shuttle III & IV, which are all done facing different corners and combined are called the "Four Corners." These are followed by "Grasping the Sparrow's Tail" (Ward Off, Left & Right, Roll Back, Press, and Push), Single Whip and "Snake Creeps Down"
34. Step Up to Seven Stars
35. Retreat to Ride Tiger
36. Turn Body, Sweep Lotus Leg
37. Bend Bow, Shoot Tiger. This posture is followed by Step Up, Block, Parry and Punch then Apparent Close-up, and lastly Cross Hands, which leads to the close of the Tai Chi form

The latest development in the popularization of Tai Chi Chuan occurred in 1956 when the Chinese government commissioned the Chinese Sports Committee to convene a panel of four Tai Chi teachers to design a simplified form of Tai Chi as exercise for the people. The result is the "24 Tai Chi Form," which gives the beginner an introduction to the essential elements of Tai Chi Chuan and needs only between four to eight minutes to complete. Although officially titled the "24 Tai Chi Form," the style actually consists of 30 named postures.

The 24 Tai Chi Form is the style used for competition and is currently believed to be the most popular form, not only in China but all over the world.

The 24 Tai Chi Form
1. Commencing
2. Part the Wild Horse's Mane
3. White Crane Spreads Its Wings
4. Brush Knee and Step Forward
5. Play the Pipa
6. Step Back and Repulse Monkey
7. Grasp Bird's Tail, Left, followed by Ward Off, Roll Back, Press and Push
8. Grasp Bird's Tail, Right
9. Single Whip
10. Wave Hands Like Clouds
11. Single Whip
12. High Pat on Horse
13. Right Heel Kick
14. Strike to Ears with Both Fists
15. Left Heel Kick
16. Snake Creeps Down and Golden Rooster Stands on One Leg, Left
17. Snake Creeps Down and Golden Rooster Stands on One Leg, Right
18. Fair Lady Works the Shuttles
19. Pick Up Needle from the Bottom of the Sea
20. Fan Penetrates Back
21. Turn Body, Deflect, Parry and Punch
22. Appears Closed (Rufeng Sibi), Withdraw and Push as if Closing a Door
23. Cross Hands (Shizishou)
24. Closing (Shoushi)

"The form of Tai Chi you choose to practise is not important," I told my listeners. "What *is* vital is that you practise Tai Chi." For more information on Tai Chi Chuan, please go online and see *www.dotaichi.com* or *www.chebucto.ns.ca.*

There was a final question. "What about breathing? I've heard that 'correct' breathing is essential to maximize the benefits of Tai Chi but I have also been told that what is 'correct' is still being defined. What do you think?" the same woman asked.

"Breathing is an important component of Tai Chi but the best respiratory technique remains to be determined. Some Tai Chi masters emphasize specific breathing patterns closely correlated with particular movements that are probably difficult for most students to follow, while many others teach a more tolerant inhale-exhale-when-you-please breathing method that is easier to practise. I personally favour the simple breath-in-with-opening movement and breath-out-with-closing when performing Tai Chi Healthercise. As a general rule, the initiation of a particular posture is the opening movement and the completion of the form is the closing action," I had told her.

My reminiscence was cut off there.

"Hello? Dr. Patrick Patience here," said a panting voice into the telephone receiver at my ear.

Say Yes to Exercise!

- Physical exercise is the ultimate panacea
- Any amount of exercise is healthy
- The best exercise is that which you enjoy
- Tai Chi Chuan is probably the perfect healthercise.

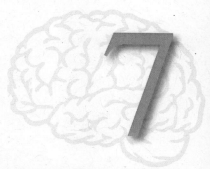

staying slim strikes strokes

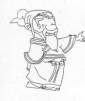

*"He who takes medicine and neglects to diet
wastes the skill of his doctors."*

~ CHINESE PROVERB

I quickly asked the emergency room charge nurse to listen in on the extension and document the time and date before speaking into the mouthpiece of the phone. "Dr. Patience, this is Dr. Felix Veloso. I'm a neurologist in Regina and I'm sorry to tell you that your father Victor suffered a stroke about 90 minutes ago," I said.

"Oh no!" he said, worry clear in his tone as he caught his breath. "Has he been treated?"

I hoped we would be able to, very soon. "We have—at most—only about another 90 minutes to complete an assessment of your father's eligibility for treatment using a recently approved blood clot buster that may save his life," I told him, "but your father says that he doesn't understand the consent form and wants us to get your approval to treat instead. He has confidence in your decision and he'll agree to whatever you decide," I added.

"You're talking about tPA," Dr. Patience replied. "I've read the research of Dr. Henrik Stig Jørgensen, which found that even if all stroke patients arrived at the hospital within the three-hour window for tPA to be safely administered, only one in 25 will gain any benefit from the blood clot-buster and that treatment with tPA may benefit single patients but will have no impact on the general prognosis of stroke.[73]

"I'm also aware that suggestions have been made to expand the three-hour window in which tPA can be safely administered[a] to 4.5 hours from ischemic stroke onset,[74] but I want you to strictly follow the three-hour, FDA-approved and research proven guideline in administering tPA to my father. Make sure he fulfills all the eligibility criteria. If he does, you have my consent to administer tPA to my dad. And please tell Dad and Mom that I'll be taking the next available flight to Regina," Dr. Patience said.

After thanking him for his confidence and confirming with the emergency room charge nurse that she had documented the time and date of Dr. Patience's telephone consent in her nursing progress notes, I hung up the phone and rushed to Radiology, holding in my hand the list of criteria for tPA treatment. In Radiology, I found the anxious, elderly, overweight and almost totally bald Victor Patience. Even prone on the X-ray table, his left-sided paralysis was obvious.

I greeted him and introduced myself. "Victor Patience? I'm Dr. Veloso. I'll be taking care of you. Don't worry; we're going to do our best for you. I just finished talking to your son Patrick and he has given his consent for us to proceed with tPA to treat your stroke. But we must first assess your eligibility for receiving the blood clot-buster safely," I reassured the distressed man, then quickly reviewed the formidable list of criteria for tPA in the acute treatment of stroke. Mr. Patience would be excluded from receiving the blood clot-buster if he met even a single one of conditions mentioned in the list:

a With acceptable risk of the serious complications of hemorrhage.

FACTORS PREVENTING tPA TREATMENT

- Onset of symptoms or the last time the patient was known to be well is greater than three hours.
- Rapidly improving neurological signs or minimal deficit. If the stroke symptoms are minimal or rapidly improving, then the patient may be having a *transient ischemic attack (TIA)* or "warning stroke" in which case tPA is not indicated
- Massive stroke with coma, *fixed eye deviation* and complete hemiplegia[b]
- CAT scan evidence of cerebral hemorrhage
- Clinical presentation consistent with *subarachnoid hemorrhage* even if CAT scan normal
- Elevated blood pressure of 185/110 and not treatable
- Blood glucose of less than three or more than 22 mmol/L
- Use of *anticoagulants,* such as *warfarin,* in previous 48 hours
- Platelet count of less than 100,000
- Internal bleeding, like gastrointestinal or urinary bleeding, within past three weeks
- History of *intracranial hemorrhage, arteriovenous malformation[c]* or *aneurysm*
- Previous stroke, major head trauma or intracranial surgery within past three months
- Recent *arterial puncture* at non-compressible site
- Major surgery within 14 days
- *Lumbar puncture* within 7 days
- *Seizures* at onset of stroke
- Myocardial infarction[d] within three weeks
- *Pericarditis[e]* within three months

b Paralysis of one side of the body.
c An abnormal connection between veins and arteries
d Heart attack.
e An inflammation of the pericardium, or sac surrounding the heart.

- Pregnancy
- Age 18 years or younger

Is it any wonder that only one of 25 stroke victims who manages to reach a hospital within three hours of stroke onset—a major accomplishment in itself—would benefit from tPA?

A careful neurological examination revealed that Mr. Victor Patience's *National Institute of Health Stroke Scale (NIHSS)* score was 15, which meant that his stroke was of moderate severity. The **NIHSS** is a 15-item neurological examination scale for stroke, used to measure several aspects of brain function, including consciousness, speech, vision, eye movement, motor strength, coordination and sensation. An experienced examiner should be able to rate the NIHSS of a stroke patient in 10 minutes or less. Ratings for each item are scored with three to five grades, with zero as normal. A maximum score of 42 represents a massive stroke from which the victim rarely recovers. An NIHSS of four or less indicates a minor stroke and suggests that tPA is not needed, whereas an NIHSS score equal to or greater than 21 signifies a severe stroke with the attendant excessive risk of serious bleeding complications from tPA treatment. Mr. Patience's NIHSS score of 15 determined that he was an ideal candidate for treatment with tPA, provided he fulfilled all of the other eligibility criteria.

"What does the CAT scan show?" I asked Dr. Emerge, who was inspecting the images in the viewing box.

"Looks fine to me. I don't see any hemorrhage. I don't see any signs of stroke, either."

I was surprised. "Come and see for yourself," he said.

After carefully examining the black and white pictures, I pointed out a spot of increased density in the first segment of the left middle cerebral artery of Mr. Patience's CAT scan.

"Dr. Emerge, this white area of increased density in M1 of the middle cerebral artery on non-contrast head CT is known as the *hyperdense middle cerebral artery sign* and is one of the earliest and most useful signs of an intra-arterial blood clot causing ischemic stroke," I explained to the emergency room physician.

"We must return Mr. Patience to the emergency department for tPA administration, stat!" I looked at my watch. "It is now 9 a.m. We have only one hour left to prepare Mr. Patience for the disability-preventing treatment."

The nurse helped Dr. Emerge and I move the hefty patient from the CAT scan table to the stretcher.

"Does anybody know how much Mr. Patience weighs?" I asked. "We need to know his exact weight in order to administer the correct dose of tPA," I added.

The recommended dose of tPA in the treatment of adult acute ischemic stroke is 0.9 mg/kg (to a maximum of 90 mg) infused over 60 minutes, with 10% of the total dose administered as an initial IV *bolus* over one minute.[f]

"We haven't had a chance to weigh him yet," the nurse replied. "Because he's paralysed on the left side we'll need a bed scale to weigh him—he's likely too heavy for an upright scale anyway," she added.

"Let's hurry up, then," I said. "We've got to get him back to ER immediately. Isn't there usually a bed scale there?"

While helping lift the overweight Mr. Patience from the CAT scan table to the stretcher, I recalled a consultation I'd had with an obese patient a year earlier.

"Good morning, Mrs. Obesitas, how may I help you?" I had asked the distressed overweight lady.

"Doctor, I have been suffering from severe back pain for at least 25 years," she said. "I have had four back operations and six MRIs over the past 10 years—the last one just six months ago. My surgeon says there is nothing more he can do for me and that I have what he called *failed back syndrome*, meaning

---

f A relatively large dose of medication administered into a vein over a short period of time.

that repeated surgery has not improved the severe, disabling back pain I feel. The pain is like a constant lightning bolt going down one or both of my legs, and I've been told I'll just have to live with it and use pain pills and patches. Pain clinics have done everything they can, too, but still I suffer! Even my chiropractor, physiotherapist, massage therapist and acupuncturist have given up on me. One of my close friends says I need another MRI, but my doctor refuses to repeat the test after the one I had six months ago failed to explain my ongoing pain."

I winced in sympathy; it sounded like torture. "How tall are you and how much do you weigh," I asked, knowing that another MRI would likely do nothing to help her back problems.

"I'm 5 feet 4 inches tall and weighed 250 pounds last time I checked three months ago," she replied.

Considering her medium-sized body frame, it was clear that Mrs. Obesitas was at least 100 pounds overweight.

"Do you know what your ideal weight is?" I asked.

She thought about it. "I figure my ideal weight should be somewhere between 125 to 140 pounds—but what has that got to do with my back? I know I'm too heavy for my height—I've been trying to lose these extra pounds since my third and last child was born 25 years ago. Come to think of it, that's when my back pain started too.

"I've tried all sorts of diets over the years, but nothing's really worked. Oh, sometimes I lose a few pounds to begin with, but then I just gain them all back and then some. I've also tried diet pills but was scared off by reports of their serious side effects. I was a waitress before I got married and never had a weight problem then. Or back pain either, even though I was on my feet 10 hours a day. Isn't that funny? You'd think I'd have had more back problems then than now when I"ve been home looking after the kids. Why is that, Dr. Veloso? Is being overweight to blame for my back pain?"

I nodded. "I believe that your obesity is not only the major cause of your persistent back pain but—if left uncorrected—may eventually lead to stroke by way of hypertension, diabetes mellitus and *dyslipidemia*,[g] all recognized high risk factors for stroke."

"I guess it's no wonder my blood pressure is still high in spite of the three different kinds of blood pressure pills I take, and my diabetes is poorly controlled, even with the two types of tablets I take. My last test showed my cholesterol levels were still elevated despite taking cholesterol-lowering medications that cause my muscles to ache all over," the dismayed lady lamented loudly. "But why have I gained so much weight when I eat basically the same amount of food a day now as I did while I was waitressing?"

I explained to Mrs. Obesitas that her back pain had made her less active—carrying around her post-pregnancy weight 25 years earlier had caused her first back pains and so she wasn't very active, which in turn caused her to gain more weight. It's a vicious cycle: the heavier she became, the more back pain she suffered; the more back pain she experienced, the more she limited her activity; the more she limited her activity, the more weight she gained because the calories she used to spend in physical activities are now being stored as body fat. I reminded Mrs. Obesitas that the formulas for the recommended caloric intake to maintain weight in an adult are:

FORMULAS FOR CALORIE INTAKE

- for **sedentary** people:
  Weight x 13 = estimated calories/day
- for **moderately active** people:
  Weight x 17 = estimated calories/day
- for **highly active** people:
  Weight x 20 = estimated calories/day

Notice that the caloric intake is directly proportional to the

g An abnormal amount of lipids (fat and/or cholesterol) in the bloodstream.

degree of physical activity. The more active you are, the more calories you need to maintain a constant weight and vice versa. If you eat more calories than you expend in physical activity, the extra calories will be stored as fat in your body and you gain weight. If you eat fewer calories than you spend in physical activity, the energy your body needs is obtained by transforming your stored fat to calories and you lose weight. You might remember from high school physics that the law of the conservation of energy states that the total amount of energy in an isolated system (in this case, your body) remains constant.

A consequence of this law is that energy cannot be created or destroyed. The only thing that can happen with energy in an isolated system is that it can change form, for instance, from chemical to thermal energy. Because energy is associated with mass in Einstein's theory of relativity, the conservation of energy also implies the conservation of mass in isolated systems. In other words, the mass of a system cannot change so long as energy is not permitted to enter or leave the system.

Conversely, mass will increase if more energy (calories) enters than exits and vice versa. Translated into living organisms, energy input (food calories) = energy output (activities of daily living + weight + exercise). This is a law of nature. It is unchangeable.

To state it in another way, the only way to lose weight (mass) is to either reduce your caloric intake or to increase your caloric output, specifically by exercising. No, ifs, ands, buts or maybes about this natural law. While she was waitressing, Mrs. Obesitas was highly active. Her caloric input was equal to her energy output and her weight remained stable. When she became a full-time homemaker, she was not as active but was probably still consuming the same—if not more—daily calories, generating an excess of calories, which were then transformed to fat and stored in her body.

This is true for all living organisms. It is well known that gorillas in the wild have to actively forage for their natural plant food and grow to a maximum weight of about 450 pounds. Gorillas caged in zoos with limited room to roam lead much more sedentary lives and grow to around 600 pounds—about a third heavier than their freely roaming cousins. The sedentary zoo gorillas are also fed highly refined, processed foods that probably contribute to the difference in weight between them and their leaner, active cousins.[75]

There are many studies that show that our Western diet, which consists mostly of refined, processed foods, is responsible for the increase in chronic degenerative diseases such as obesity and diabetes, but the most persuasive is the 1992 research involving 10 Australian Aborigines living a sedentary lifestyle in urban settlements in Western Australia. They developed obesity, diabetes mellitus, hypertension and dyslipidemia from eating the highly refined, processed foods typical of the Western diet. The obese, hypertensive and diabetic Aborigines participated in an experiment in which they agreed to return to their natural habitat in the bush where they had to forage for natural plants and hunt wild game to eat. Professor Kerin O'Dea, director of Sansom Institute of Health Research of the Health Sciences Divisional Office, University of South Australia, the nutritionist who conducted the research, found that all 10 subjects not only lost a significant amount of weight, but more importantly, their diabetes and dyslipidemia vanished and their high blood pressure normalized after they had returned to their original natural lifestyle for just seven weeks.[76]

"Dr. Veloso, you've talked about calories, but I still don't have a clear idea of what they are. How are they related to energy?" asked Mrs. Obesitas.

"A **calorie** is a unit of thermal energy usually used in diet plans and on nutrition labels to determine the amount of energy that food provides," I informed Mrs. Obesitas.

"All right. With all this talk of diets, do you have a recommendation for how I should change my eating habits?" she asked, now greatly motivated.

"Sure!" I said. "The My Slow Plant Meal."

- **My:** This diet belongs to you. It is your plan and you design your own regimen and you are responsible for the success of the diet.

- **Slow:** Eating slowly allows for the estimated 20 minutes for the sensation of fullness signaled by your stomach to reach your brain so that you know to stop eating. Taking time to relish your food will prevent you from overeating.

  Researchers have identified a chemical messenger called *N-acylphosphatidylethanolamine* (NAPE).[77] Secreted by the small intestine after a meal, it takes approximately 20 minutes to signal the satiety centre in your brain to stop eating. Take the time to enjoy the flavours and taste of your food. You have worked hard to earn, buy and prepare your food. You deserve to leisurely enjoy the fruits of your labour.

- **Plant:** Plants are the healthiest of foods because vegetation gets its vitality for existence directly from the sun—the ultimate source of energy that fuels all life on Earth. You might recall from high school biology that green plants and micro-organisms such as algae convert sunlight energy into chemical energy in a process call *photosynthesis* that transforms carbon dioxide, water and light into organic compounds, particularly carbohydrates and oxygen. Plants store this chemical energy in their leaves and seeds for use as needed. Plants use the carbohydrates to make fats and proteins, which are stored in their leaves, stems and seeds. Only green plants containing chlorophyll are capable of photosynthesis and are therefore the sole sources of food that animals depend on to survive. All foods originate directly or indirectly from the photosynthetic ability of plants. Plants contain all the macro and micronutrients needed to sustain life.

When humans eat meat, we are really eating plants that are transformed into flesh by *herbivorous* (plant-eating) animals. But only 10% of the energy in plants is transformed into meat by the herbivores. The remaining 90% of the plant food energy is used in metabolic activities to keep the animal alive. In other words, it takes 10 pounds of vegetation to produce one pound of meat.[78] What a waste of precious, life-sustaining food! Even more concerning is the fact that the process of changing plant food to meat likely entails some loss of essential micronutrients—particularly phytochemicals—and also alters the quality of the macronutrients (proteins, carbohydrates and fats) by adding, or increasing the amounts of, harmful fats in the animal meat.

A prime example of this biological effect is the feeding of processed grains to cattle penned in feedlots for the purpose of fattening the animal. This has the unintended and possibly harmful effect of increasing the proportion of *omega-6* to *omega-3* fatty acids in the animal's fat. Another illustration of the harmful effects of transforming plant to animal foods is the change in composition of the *amino acids* in their proteins so that animal proteins have higher contents of *lysine* and *methionine*,[h] which are known to produce *hypercholesterolemia.*[i] In contrast, plant proteins have greater amounts of *arginine,* which has the opposite effect of lowering cholesterol.[79] In addition, the higher up in the food chain pyramid the organism feeds, the greater are its risks of eating an increasing amount of toxic chemicals such as *DDT, dioxin* and *mercury* that accumulate in lower level consumers. And humans eat at the very top of the food chain pyramid!

- **Meal:** The word *meal* connotes the fine art of dining on highly nutritious yet low-calorie, lovingly prepared, foods at dedicated times of the day. Not all foods are created equal; some are better quality with a higher nutrient value and lower calories, while some have fewer nutrients and pack more calories although they weigh the same. Check the label!

One hundred grams of vegetable oil contains 884 calories while the same amount of iceberg lettuce has only 13. One hundred grams of roast beef contains 280 calories and supplies 21 grams of protein, yet 100 grams of tofu has less than a quarter of the calories—only 73!—but provides more than one-third the protein at 8 grams. It is easy to calculate that you ingest more than three times the amount of calories by eating a similar quantity of oil compared to beef, and about 12 times more calories compared to eating an equal amount of tofu. What is even more worrisome is that there is zero amount of tissue-building protein in the 884 calories of 100 grams of oil.

---

h Two essential amino acids.
i A high level of cholesterol in the blood, which is a precursor to many forms of disease, particularly those of the heart.

Eat three meals a day—breakfast, lunch and supper. Three daily meals provide a stable supply of energy to let you perform at maximum efficiency throughout the day and prevent wide fluctuations of blood sugar that may lead to binge eating from *hypoglycemia.*[j] Three meals a day also fit best with most of our work schedules. Refrain but do not completely abstain from snacks. If you like to munch—and who doesn't?—just limit your refreshments to fruits and vegetables. As much as you like. In fact, the more vegetables and fruits you eat, the more weight you will lose.

Mrs. Obesitas had listened intently. "Am I hearing right? Did you say that the more vegetables and fruits I eat, the more weight I will lose? How can I eat more and weigh less?" she asked, puzzled. "Surely you must be mistaken, Dr. Veloso!"

"There's no mistake," I said. "Yes, you can eat more and yet weigh less if you consume foods with a negative thermic effect." I assured her. "All foods have a caloric cost to chewing, digesting and absorbing them, an expense known as the *thermic effect* or *specific dynamic action,* in other words, the calories expended by our bodies to eat and digest the foods we consume."

The three macronutrients in food have widely different thermic effects. **Protein** has the highest thermic effect, with estimates ranging as high as 30% of its caloric content. That means that almost one-third of the calories of ingested protein is lost in processing it, whereas the thermic effect of **fat** is—at most—3%. So 97% of the calories in ingested fat are easily stored in our bodies as fat. The thermic effect of **carbohydrates** is somewhere between those two extremes, probably at about 7% of its energy content. The low thermic effect of fat is another reason to avoid it if you want to lose weight.[80]

---

j   Low blood sugar, which may result in symptoms like sweating, trembling, hunger, dizziness, moodiness, confusion and blurred vision.

The thermic effect of vegetables and fruits, however, is about 20% and, in fact, many fibrous fruits and vegetables have a *negative* thermic effect, which means that you use more calories to process the foods than is contained in the plants themselves. For example, a stick of celery may contain five calories but you could spend up to 90 calories ingesting, digesting and assimilating it, resulting in a net energy expenditure of 85 calories, which comes from burning up the fat stores in your body.

"Vegetables and fruits must therefore definitely be a part of your diet if you are watching your weight," I told Mrs. Obesitas.

A partial list of **negative thermic effect vegetables** includes: asparagus, broccoli, cabbage, carrot, cauliflower, celery, cucumber, green beans, lettuce and spinach.

Some **negative thermic effect fruits** are apples, cranberries, grapefruit, oranges, peaches and strawberries.

"A word of caution though: do not limit your daily food intake to just negative thermic effect foods. It is always healthier to eat a variety of high nutrition low-calorie foods every day," I concluded.

"My husband believes that 'real men' eat red meat," said Mrs. Obesitas. "Are there healthy alternatives to traditional beef and pork red meats?"

Again I nodded. "Venison and bison meat from free-ranging, grass-grazing deer and buffalo are lean, low-cholesterol red meats rich in omega-3 fatty acids that any 'real man' can safely enjoy," I replied with a chuckle.

"He'll like that. I've read that individual vegetables don't contain the complete protein we need because they lack certain essential amino acids," she said.

"You're right," I agreed. "Further, vegetables are also missing *Vitamin B$_{12}$*, a vital micronutrient without which serious diseases, including dementia and paralysis, are possible.

"Please do not misunderstand me," I went on. "I am not necessarily advocating a complete vegetarian existence. I am recommending a plant-dominant diet and to eat meat—particularly red meat—*only* as a small or occasional addition to a vegetable-heavy meal, not as the main component. Remember, everything in moderation!

"But do keep in mind that consuming a mixed variety of complimentary plant foods *will* supply all eight of the essential amino acids needed by humans," I assured Mrs. Obesitas. "And would you believe that there is an inexpensive and widely available, highly nutritious, low-calorie legume that is not only a complete protein, but when fermented is also a rich source of Vitamin B_{12}?"

"Really? What is this ideal plant food?" an intrigued Mrs. Obesitas eagerly asked.

"Soybean!" I responded. "The soybean is a legume that has been used in China for 5,000 years. Soy contains significant amounts of the eight **essential amino acids**: *phenylalanine, valine, threonine, tryptophan, isoleucine, methionine, leucine* and *lysine*. The United States Food and Drug Agency considers soy protein products to be a good substitute for animal meats because it is a complete protein. And they've approved the health claim that soy protein may reduce cholesterol and the risk of heart disease."[81]

Raw soybean is difficult to digest because of its high content of *trypsin inhibitors* that prevent the breakdown of proteins. The good news is that the trypsin inhibitors in soybeans are easily destroyed by cooking. It is therefore essential that only cooked soybean products, such as *tofu*, be consumed.

Fermented tofu such as *miso* and *tempeh* are rich sources of Vitamin B_{12}. Soy is the best source of protein for vegetarians and for people who cannot afford meat. It is the nutritional equivalent of meat and eggs for human growth and health. Soybeans have the highest yield per square metre of growing area compared to other legume seeds, and are the least expensive source of dietary protein.[82]

Soybean oil is one of the few vegetable oils to contain a significant amount of omega-3 fatty acids, particularly *alpha-linolenic acid*.[83] **Omega-3 fatty acids** are special fat components that benefit many functions of the human body. Research has reported that soy protein significantly decreases cholesterol in the blood, reduces *low density lipoprotein* (LDL—bad cholesterol), lowers *triglyceride* concentration[k] and may increase *high density lipoprotein* (HDL—good cholesterol).[84] Among the conclusions reached by a panel of the American Heart Association, who reviewed the health benefits of soybeans, is the statement that "soy products such as tofu, soy butter, soy nuts, or some soy burgers should be beneficial to cardiovascular and overall health because of their high content of polyunsaturated fats, fiber, vitamins, and minerals and low content of saturated fat. Using these and other soy foods to replace foods high in animal protein that contain saturated fat and cholesterol may confer benefits to cardiovascular health."[85]

BENEFITS OF SOYBEANS

Besides preventing stroke and heart disease, soybeans offer several other health benefits, including:

- improving diabetes mellitus control
- reducing menopause symptoms
- preventing obesity.[86]

In addition, researchers report that soybeans and non-fermented soy products such as tofu contain high levels of several compounds with demonstrated anti-cancer properties—including inhibiting the growth of cancer cells.[l] Soybean consumption is

k A chain of three molecules of fatty acids combined with glycerol that form lipids (the basic water-insoluble substances that circulate in the blood). Elevated triglyceride levels are associated with the development of atheriosclerosis, heart disease and stroke.

l These compounds include phytates, protease inhibitors, phytosterols, saponins, genistein and diadzein. Winston J. Craig, Ph.D., R.D. "Phytochemicals: Guardians of Our Health." Vegetarian Nutrition. American Dietetic Association.. http://www.vegetariannutrition.net/articles/Phytochemicals-Guardians-of-Our-Health.php. Accessed October 20, 2010.

reportedly responsible for the lower incidence of breast, prostate, stomach, colon, rectal and lung cancers[87] in Chinese and Japanese men and women. One explanation for the breast cancer-preventing effect of soybean is likely because of its high content of *genistein*, which acts as an anti-estrogen agent by binding to estrogen receptors, thereby lowering the activity of *endogenous estrogen*—the female sex hormone produced by the body during menstruation—and reducing the growth of estrogen-sensitive tumours.[88]

Eating more soy and other vegetables has other benfits, too:

- Up to 16 pounds of soybeans and grain are needed to produce one pound of beef, which means that 1.3 billion human beings could be fed annually on the grains and soybeans eaten by U.S. livestock
- the 60 million people who will starve to death this year could be adequately fed by the grain saved if Americans reduced their intake of meat by 10%
- 90% of protein is wasted by cycling grain through livestock
- 20,000 pounds of potatoes can be grown on one acre of land, compared to 100 pounds of beef that can be produced on that same single acre.

Soybeans are an ideal food. Their only minor imperfection is their content of trypsin inhibitors that render the raw bean difficult to digest. However, the Chinese corrected this slight flaw by transforming soybeans into tofu, in the process converting soybeans into a most nutritious, digestible food, and making them arguably the most consumed plant of all time.

What is tofu? Like four other great Chinese inventions—paper, the compass, gunpowder and printing—the discovery of tofu is lost in the mists of China's 5,000 years of civilization, although most scholars agree that tofu was already being eaten at least 2,000 years ago. There are several hypotheses concerning the origin of tofu but the most plausible are the Accidental Coagulation Theory, which proposes that tofu was developed around 600 A.D. when pureed soybean soup was seasoned with sea water containing *magnesium sulfate*. The other, more believable speculation is the Mongolian Import Theory, which postulates that the basic method for making tofu was adapted by the Chinese from milk-drinking Mongolian tribes living along the northern border of China. But regardless of its origin, there is no doubt that tofu is a crucial source of protein in the meat-poor diet of most Chinese people and the preferred meatless meal of Buddhists.[89]

A staple in Asia, tofu is known for its extraordinary nutritional benefits, as well as its versatility. **Tofu**, also known as bean curd, is a soft cheese-like food made by curdling soy milk with a coagulant, usually *gypsum* or *calcium sulfate*. Tofu is tasteless and easily absorbs the flavours of other food ingredients. Fresh tofu is usually sold packaged in water and should be refrigerated and kept in water until used. Tofu can be kept fresh for up to a week if the water containing it is changed daily. Tofu can be frozen for up to three months, but note that freezing it will make the tofu slightly chewier. Types of tofu:

- **Firm tofu** is dense and can be stir-fried, grilled, scrambled, baked or served in soups. Firm tofu has higher protein, fat and calcium content and is most commonly used in cooking
- **Soft tofu** is usually blended with other food ingredients
- **Silken tofu** has a creamy texture and is delicious as a dessert, particularly if sweetened with honey or maple syrup
- **Dried tofu,** such as dried bean curd skin and bean curd sheet, should be rehydrated before cooking

- **Fermented tofu** has an aged cheese aroma and includes *tempeh, miso, natto* and *doufu-ru* that are usually used as condiments
- **Westernized** tofu or *textured vegetable protein (TVP)* is used to make imitation meat products such as veggie sausages, veggie burgers, veggie ground meat, veggie hot dogs and veggie bacon.

Soybeans are also processed into "dairy" foods like soy milk, soy margarine, soy ice cream, soy yogurt and soy cheese. Imitation meats and dairy products made from soy are readily available in most supermarkets. Though there has been some concern that excessive intake of soy might suppress *thyroid* function, no solid evidence has been documented to support this.

"What about liquid calories?" Mrs. Obesitas had then asked. "If our bodies are mostly water, then liquid must be a major component of our daily diet, right?"

Again I nodded. "Experts recommend drinking between 48 to 64 ounces of liquid daily, although most would agree that thirst is a better guide to our individual fluid requirements. The amount of food the average adult eats daily provides about 20% of the total daily water intake required. The remaining 80% comes from the beverages we drink. Plain water is the best beverage for meeting our daily fluid requirements.

"Regrettably, most of us satisfy our liquid needs by drinking pop, which is high in calories—most of them empty. Drinking just one regular can of pop per day adds 150 calories to our daily caloric intake, or 54,750 calories a year. Since 3500 calories equals one pound of body weight, that one-soda-a-day habit can pile on more than 15 pounds a year!" I told Mrs. Obesitas.

"And although coffee is calorie-free, most of us stir in at least one tablespoon of cream—which has more than 50 calories—and/or one tablespoon of sugar—which adds almost another 50 calories—for a total of 100 calories in one regular cup of coffee.

So consuming just one regular cup of café au lait daily can add up to a pound of extra body weight monthly!"

She shook her head in consternation. "I usually drink two cups of coffee at breakfast and a cup during the afternoon, as well as a can of soda at lunch and supper. That adds up to ... let me see ... 500 calories daily!" She sounded shocked.

"That's about 25% of your total daily calorie requirements in beverages alone,"[m] I said, dismayed. "It all adds up to 3,500 calories or a solid pound of body weight. That's 52 pounds in a year." I hoped the message was getting through to her.

"Well, no *wonder* I continue to gain weight even when I restrict my food calories!" She thought about it for a minute then asked, "So why are liquid calories rarely emphasized in weight reduction diets?"

She had a point. "You're right, Mrs. Obesitas. And studies have even confirmed that liquid calorie intake plays an equal— if not *greater*—impact on weight gain than solid calorie intake. But there *is* some good news. I've recently learned that of all commonly consumed beverages, **tea** not only does *not* increase weight, it may in fact reduce it! Researchers reportedly found that tea, especially green tea with its high content of the *polyphenol, catechin*, promotes *thermogenesis* by inhibiting the enzyme *catechol-O-methyl transferase (COMT)*, which degrades *noradrenadine* and thus allows the sympathetic hormone to prolong its action of burning fatty acid to generate energy, resulting in weight loss."

Mrs. Obesitas was paying close attention.

The most romantic version of the origin of tea is that a Buddhist monk, trying to stay awake to continue praying, cut off his eyelids. The cast-away eyelids took root and grew into a tea bush. The most historically credible account is that the second emperor of China, Shen Nung, discovered tea in 2737 B.C. when leaves from the tea plant, *Camellia sinensis*, accidentally

---

m Assuming a daily intake of 2,000 calories.

blew into his cup of hot water, which he drank boiled for sanitary reasons. Emperor Shen Nung found the golden yellow brew to be most refreshing and encouraged his subjects to adapt a similar healthy practice of drinking the leaves steeped in boiled water. Upon hearing that the famous sage Lu-Yu in 780 A.D. praised tea as the "Dew of Heaven," Shen Nung, decided that he, as the emperor and "Son of Heaven," deserved to drink only the finest "Dew of Heaven" and issued a royal edict ordering that the best tea from the four corners of his kingdom be sent as a tribute to the Forbidden City for the imperial court to enjoy.[90]

During the Tang Dynasty (618-907 A.D.), Tang Xuan Zong asked a monk renowned to be more than 130 years old his secret for long life. The aged monk answered: "Drink tea daily, nothing else." And so tea as a health tonic was established. The medicinal supremacy bestowed upon tea by Traditional Chinese Medicine (TCM) is evidenced by its counsel: "Better to go without food for three days than without tea for a single day." Practitioners of this ancient healing art continue to preach what Western medicine is increasingly discovering: "food is medicine and medicine is food." Clearly, TCM recognized tea as a panacea early on and has long recommended particular teas for specific health indications:

- **Green or Jasmine tea:**
  - as an antioxidant to remove *free radicals* in the human body
  - to reduce blood sugar
  - to reduce the harmful effects of smoking
  - to prevent and reduce cancer growth
  - to prevent allergies, cold and flu
  - to promote oral hygiene, including prevention of cavities

- **Black or Pu'erh tea:**
    - to reduce the risk of heart disease
    - to reduce arthritis
    - to prevent osteoporosis
    - to relieve fatigue
    - to relieve stress
- **Pu'erh or Jasmine tea:**
    - to reduce the risk of blood clots
    - to maintain fluid balance
    - to protect the liver
    - to lose weight
- **Green or Pu'erh tea** to reduce the risk of stroke
- **Pu'erh or Tuocha tea** to reduce bad cholesterol in the blood
- **Jasmine tea** to reduce high blood pressure and enhance immunity
- **Black tea** to increase alertness.[91]

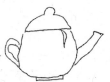

In addition to Traditional Chinese medical beliefs, tea connoisseurs credit the popularity of tea to its many health benefits:

BENEFITS OF DRINKING TEA

- Tea contains fluoride that protects teeth against cavities
- Tea has antibacterial properties that prevent *gingivitis* and associated *halitosis* (bad breath)
- Tea reduces arthritis
- Tea prevents osteoporosis
- Tea prevents Type 1 diabetes mellitus by regulating blood glucose
- Tea reduces inflammation associated with bowel diseases like Crohn's disease and ulcerative colitis

- Tea diminishes liver damage from alcohol and liver tumour
- Tea inhibits cancer, especially of the gastrointestinal tract and bladder
- Tea reduces the incidence of death after a heart attack by up to 44%
- Tea increases immunity against viruses, particularly flu and maybe even AIDS
- Tea reduces high blood pressure by up to 50%.
- Tea dilates arteries, leading to improved cardio-vascular health[92]
- Tea protects against the development of Parkinson's disease
- Tea lowers cholesterol, particularly "bad cholesterol."[93]

Researchers from the Department of Pharmacology, Faculty of Medicine, University of Hong Kong found that Chinese green teas lower blood and liver cholesterol of diet-induced, *hypercholesterolimic* (high blood cholesterol) rats, apparently by increasing fecal cholesterol excretion.[94] Other studies show that green tea catechins inhibit oxidation of LDL cholesterol, making it less likely to cause atherosclerosis and increase levels of the good HDL cholesterol, as well as:

- ease anxiety and lighten depression
- enhance cognition and possibly delay dementia
- thin blood by inhibiting platelet aggregation
- protect skin from sunburns.[95]

How to brew the most healthful, tasty tea:

- Use loose tea leaves
- Use one teaspoon (approximately two grams) of

tea for every standard six-ounce cup, more or less according to individual tea strength preference

- Use natural spring or filtered tap water
- Let boiled water stand for about five minutes to cool down to between 70° to 90° C for white and green teas
- Brew tea for approximately two minutes for first steep of green and white teas
- Double the brewing time for subsequent steeps
- Green, white and pu'erh teas are good for three to four or more brewings
- Used nearly boiled water (90° to 100° C) to brew black and pu'erh tea for five minutes.
- Black tea should be brewed only once
- Brew tea preferably in clay or ceramic teapots to avoid the metallic taste of steel teapots
- Refrain from drinking tea infused overnight because it is less healthful
- Green, jasmine or oolong teas are better drunk after eating because they may irritate an empty stomach
- You may add honey to sweeten the bitterness of over-brewed green tea
- You may add milk to black or pu'erh tea but NOT to green or oolong tea
- Used tea leaves need not necessarily be thrown away. Tea is so versatile it can even be useful after repeated steeping. Dried brewed tea leaves (also known as *chagra*) maybe employed as:
  - Fertilizer in your garden or flower pot
  - Carpet cleaner: sprinkle chagra in carpet and let sit for a few minutes before vacuuming to deodorize and sanitize carpets
  - Deodorizer: loose, dry, brewed tea can be used

as cat litter or in a thin cotton bag placed in the refrigerator or garbage can to eliminate odours
- For the adventurous, brewed tea leaves are edible and may be added to soups, vegetable dishes or salads to fully use all its goodness.

"No wonder tea is the most popular beverage in the world after water!" I told Mrs. Obesitas. "It is estimated that 18-20 billion 6 oz. cups of tea are drunk daily on our planet!"

I told Mrs. Obesitas that although all teas from China originate from the *Camellia sinensis* plant, it's the processing of the leaves after harvesting that produces the four main types of Chinese teas:

- **White**: White teas are the least processed of any tea and therefore taste the most like fresh leaves. White teas are reputed to have the highest antioxidant properties. White teas most sought after by tea drinkers are *Bai Hao Yin Zhen* (Silver Needle) and *Bai Mu Dan* (White Peony).

- **Green**: Green teas, like white, are not fermented. The plucked tea leaves are laid out to wither for about eight to 24 hours, and are steamed or pan-fried to destroy the oxidative enzymes responsible for fermentation. Favourite green teas include *Lung Ching* (Dragon Well) and *gunpowder* (Pearl).

- **Oolong**: Oolong teas are partially fermented. The plucked tea leaves are laid out to wither for about eight to 24 hours, just like in the processing of green teas, but are then tossed in baskets to bruise the edges of the leaves and thereby liberate some of the oxidative enzymes that cause the leaves to partially ferment. The leaves are then steamed to neutralize the enzymes and stop further oxidation. The most popular oolong tea is *Ti Kuan Yin*, named after the Buddhist goddess of mercy.

- **Black**: Black teas are fully fermented. The plucked tea leaves are laid out to wither for about eight to 24 hours just like in the processing of oolong tea, but unlike oolong, tea leaves destined to be black are rolled in order to break open the leaf surface so that the complete complement of oxidative enzymes will be exposed to the air for total fermentation to occur. This turns the tea black. Famous Chinese black teas include *Keemun,* which connoisseurs refer to as the "burgundy of teas" and Pu'erh.

- **Compressed (brick) tea**: Tea leaves are compressed and hardened into different shapes, especially bricks, giving it this nickname. Brick tea is ideal for transport to ethnic minorities living in the border areas of China. Compressed tea is black in colour and is therefore known in China as "black tea."

- **Scented tea** is a blend of tea leaves and fresh sweet flowers. Favourites include jasmine- and chrysanthemum-blended teas.

- **Herbal tea** or *tisane* is an infusion made from anything other than the leaves of the tea bush, *Camellia sinensis,* and include such favourites as *chamomile, peppermint* and *rosehip.*

- **Popular non-Chinese black teas** include:
  - *Assam,* grown in northeastern India, is the most

famous Indian tea. It is a strong tea with a malty
and full bodied taste. Breakfast tea is often Assam.

° *Darjeeling*, from the foothills of the Himalayas,
is often called the "champagne of teas." It has a
delicate taste.

° Sri Lanka's *Kenilworth* tea is called a "self-drinker"
because it is unblended and is among the world's
favourites for having a clean, bright flavour.[96]

Mrs. Obesitas had been listening avidly. But suddenly something occurred to her. "It seems that everything has a negative side effect, surely tea is no exception. Are there any down sides to drinking tea?"

"The health benefits of drinking tea far outweigh the possible side effects of excessive tea consumption," I told her. "Still, you should know that:

• there are very rare reports of liver problems from concentrated green tea extracts but not green tea beverages

• tea contains caffeine, which can cause insomnia, anxiety, irritability, upset stomach, nausea, diarrhea, or frequent urination in some people. It is important to realize that the strongest tea has less than 50% of the caffeine content of the weakest coffee. The average 8 oz. cup of green tea contains anywhere from 8 to 20 mg. of caffeine, while black tea contains between 40 to 60 mg. An 8 oz. cup of drip coffee has about 90 to 150 mg. It would take at least four cups of the strongest green tea to equal the caffeine content of the weakest drip coffee. The recommended caffeine consumption for an average adult is 200 mg. per day

- tea contains small amounts of *Vitamin K*, which can interact with anticoagulant drugs such as warfarin, making the drug less effective. You should have a blood clotting test known as an *international normalized ratio (INR)* test done often to correct for this imbalance if you are taking blood thinners."[97]

"While we're on the subject of healthful beverages," she said, "I have heard that **cocoa** has as much as *three* times the amount of antioxidants as tea.[98] And I love chocolate! Yet, I've been avoiding it because I'm overweight. Can I get any of chocolate's health benefits without gaining more weight?" the obese lady inquired, her voice lifting hopefully.

I nodded. "It's true—cocoa has many health benefits."

BENEFITS OF DRINKING COCOA

- Cocoa lowers blood pressure
- Cocoa improves circulation by relaxing blood vessels
- Cocoa prevents *platelet aggregation*—an essential step in blood clotting—thereby preventing heart attack and stroke
- Cocoa has a high content of *flavonoids*, powerful antioxidants that neutralize free radicals and prevent cellular damage that can lead to chronic diseases such as cancer, heart disease, stroke and high blood pressure.[99]

"But to avoid the weight gain side effect of chocolate, it is important to differentiate between *hot cocoa*, a beverage prepared from powder made by extracting most of the rich cocoa butter out of ground cacao beans, from *hot chocolate,* which is made directly from chocolate bars containing cocoa, sugar and cocoa butter. The main difference between hot cocoa and hot chocolate is the latter's richness of cocoa butter. The absence of cocoa butter makes hot cocoa *significantly* lower in caloric content and therefore much less fattening, while still preserving all the goodness of chocolate. When it comes to chocolate bars, choose the dark variety and avoid high-calorie milk chocolate, since the addition of milk and sugar dilutes and negates the health benefits of cocoa beans. The caffeine content of chocolate should not be an issue since it is less than 10% of that of coffee."[100]

Mrs. Obesitas had one last question. "Dr. Veloso, I know that wholesome nutrients help to avoid strokes, but is there any scientific evidence that a healthy diet prevents hardening of the arteries?"

Again I nodded. "You would be interested to know that:

- researchers reported in the results of a two-year study of 322 participants in the Dietary Intervention to Reverse Carotid Atherosclerosis trial that healthy foods, including either low-fat, Mediterranean or low-carbohydrate diets can induce a significant regression of *carotid vessel wall volume* (a measurement of atherosclerosis).[101] Previous investigations have found that a healthy lifestyle can stop the progression of carotid atherosclerosis, but I believe this is the only report that a healthy diet not only arrests but can actually *reduce* atherosclerosis.

- a study of 6,113 adult participants in the National Health and Nutrition Examination Survey (NHANES) from 1999 to 2006 found that subjects who consumed food with higher levels of sugar showed an elevated risk of as much as 300% reduced levels of good HDL cholesterol. The American Heart

Association has advised adults to cut added sugar to roughly five teaspoons (80 calories worth or 5% of daily calories) for women and nine teaspoons (144 calories) for men. One teaspoon of sugar equals four grams or 16 calories," I informed Mrs. Obesitas.[102]

"It seems there is compelling evidence that the three Ts—Tai Chi Chuan, Tea and Tofu—are responsible for the fact that China has one of the lowest rates of stroke in the world!" I finished.

These memories were interrupted by the nurse's disturbing report: "Dr. Veloso! We cannot weigh Mr. Patience because the bed scale is missing from the ER."

Food is Medicine

- Reach your ideal weight by balancing calorie input against energy output
- Lose weight by reducing calorie intake and/or increasing the frequency, duration and intensity of physical activities
- Gain weight by eating more calories and/or moderating physical activities
- Avoid sodas
- Drink tea
- Snack on fruits and vegetables
- Add soybean products to your diet
- Maximize the amount of plant and whole grain foods in your meals
- Choose hot cocoa over chocolate milk, and dark chocolate instead of light chocolate.

8

normalizing hypertension neutralizes strokes

 Studies show that high blood pressure is the most significant known risk factor for stroke.

We rushed Victor Patience back to emergency as soon as Dr. Emerge, two nurses and I transferred him from the X-ray bed to the stretcher.

"Quick, where is the bed scale?" I asked Florence, the stroke nurse, who met us as we returned to the ER.

"In the Stroke Care Unit (SCU). It was taken over there early this morning to weigh a stroke victim admitted late last night," Florence said.

"Please rush Mr. Patience to treatment room one and start another IV but leave him on the stretcher for now. We must weigh him as soon as I reclaim the bed scale from SCU before transferring him to a bed for tPA."

On my way to SCU, I rushed by Dr. Critico, the intensivist,[a] who had apparently been alerted by Florence of the possibility of emergency tPA treatment.

"Where's the stroke patient?" Dr. Critico asked.

---

a A physician specializing in intensive medical care.

"In ER treatment room one, but please come with me to SCU to retrieve the bed scale; we need to weigh the patient so we can determine the correct dose of tPA to safely administer," I panted.

We found the bed scale parked by the nursing desk in SCU.

"May I take the scale back to ER?" I asked the charge nurse.

"Yes, Dr. Veloso. It's been waiting for the porter to pick up for the past two hours," she said.

Having retrieved the scale, Dr. Critico and I waited for what seemed like an eternity before the elevator reached our floor. When the doors opened, we thrust the bed scale inside. Charging out of the elevator, we nearly ran into Mrs. Patience in our sprint to the ER. I agreed to her request to be with her husband in the treatment room.

"Dr. Veloso, his blood pressure is 220/140," Florence called out as soon as she saw me. The highest blood pressure for safe administration of tPA in acute stroke is 185/110.

"How can we bring down his BP fast?" I asked Dr. Critico.

"*Labetalol*—a beta-blocker that also inhibits *alpha-adrenergic receptors*[b] and safely lowers blood pressure rapidly, usually within about five minutes—is my preferred treatment for hypertensive emergencies. I would recommend an IV bolus of 20 mg of labetalol over two minutes, followed by an infusion of 0.5 to 2 mg per minute, or 20 to 80 mg every 10 minutes. In my experience, BP is almost always lowered to the desired level in less than 30 minutes with this regimen," Dr. Critico responded.

I asked Dr. Critico to proceed with the labetalol treatment without delay while helping move Mr. Patience onto the bed scale.

"He weighs 104.5 kg, about 230 lbs," Florence announced,

---

b A receptor in cell membranes sensitive to the sympathetic adrenaline and noradrenaline hormones. Stimulation of alpha-adrenergic receptors increases blood pressure and inhibition of the receptors lowers blood pressure. Labetalol blocks the binding of adrenaline to alpha-adrenergic receptors and rapidly lowers blood pressure.

"and he's about 5 feet 8 inches tall. I estimate he's about 34 kgs or 76 lbs overweight."

It is crucial to know the stroke patient's weight to give him the research-proven effective safe dose of tPA of 0.9 mg/kg—up to a maximum of 90 mg—with 10% of the dose in an IV bolus, the remainder infused over one hour. I asked Florence to prepare the maximum dose of 90 mg of tPA to be given to Mr. Patience as soon as his BP was lowered to less than 180/110 and he was otherwise assessed to fulfill all the other eligibility criteria for tPA treatment of acute ischemic stroke.

Dr. Critico started the labetalol infusion as soon as we transferred Mr. Patience back to the treatment bed.

"TRAUMA ALERT, 20 MINUTES. TRAUMA ALERT, 20 MINUTES" boomed the public address system. Apparently at least one serious injury in a major motor vehicle accident was being ambulanced to the hospital. I glanced quickly at the wall clock and realized that the accident victim would arrive at about the same time that the three-hour window for Mr. Patience to benefit from tPA ended. The accident victim's arrival would stress the emergency room's scarce resources. It was now critical that Mr. Patience receive tPA before the trauma arrived so that both of these emergencies could receive the maximum benefits of the hospital's limited resources.

The race against time had intensified.

Turning again to Mrs. Patience, I asked her if she knew her husband's blood pressure was dangerously elevated.

She answered that he had had hypertension for many years and was on medication that he took irregularly. The side effects of these drugs (coughing and frequent urination) kept him awake at night, so he often skipped taking the medications. "If only there was something he could have done without drugs, his blood pressure wouldn't be so high," she lamented.

Checking the time once more, I told Mrs. Patience about Mr. Harper Tencion.

It had been a blizzardy Saskatchewan winter morning two years earlier when Mr. Harper Tencion requested an urgent appointment. He was a successful, middle-aged restauranteur with a stocky build and his idea of exercise was the once-a-week 50-metre walk from his bank's parking lot to the teller wicket to deposit the restaurant's income. He loved eating the creamy cuisines prepared by the award-winning chefs in his bistro. I once commented that the meals served in his restaurant were too salty and would be healthier if they were lower in *sodium* content. Mr. Tencion retorted that Canadians crave salty food, and that he would go broke and lose his only excuse to exercise once a week if his restaurant served only low-salt fare.

A survey by the World Action on Salt and Health (WASH) of over 260 food products available around the world from several international fast food processors revealed that Canadian versions of these foods had higher levels of salt compared to most other countries. The food processors' reported explanation for the high sodium content of their Canadian products was that they satisfied "Canadians' demand for salty foods"—a justification consistent with Mr. Tencion's rationale.[103]

Mr. Tencion was also a migraine-sufferer whose headaches had been successfully aborted by a *triptan* medication[c] as needed for several years.

"Thank you for seeing me," he said after our customary greeting of "Good morning," even as the gusting wind outside my warm office howled against the angry sky, still dark at 10 a.m.

"What's happened?" I wanted to know. "When I last saw you, you were doing fine and your annual check-up isn't until next year. Why are you here so much earlier?"

"Well, Dr. Veloso, shortly after I saw you six months ago, I was diagnosed with high blood pressure by my family doctor, who prescribed several medications—all of which I discontin-

---

c A type of medication used to treat migraines and cluster headaches.

ued after a few weeks because of their intolerable side effects. I suffered a whole range of them!"

I felt badly for Mr. Tencion, knowing that these side effects could include fatigue, depression, slow heart rate, low blood potassium, palpitations, constipation, worse headaches, coughing, frequent urination, impotence, dizziness and drowsiness.

I explained to him that **high blood pressure** is:

- defined as a *systolic* blood pressure of 140 mmHg or higher, or a *diastolic* blood pressure of 90 mmHg or higher [d]
- high if it is consistently more than 140/90
- very common, affecting about 35% of all adults
- nicknamed the "silent killer" because it almost always has no symptoms
- known to increase stroke risk by four to six times
- the single most important controllable stroke risk factor. The others are smoking, lack of exercise, obesity, diabetes mellitus, alcohol/drug abuse and hypercholesterolemia (high cholesterol)
- the stroke risk factor that is the easiest to correct naturally

and that **prehypertension**:

- is a systolic blood pressure of between 120–139 over diastolic of 80–89
- affects about 15% of adults
- along with hypertension, damages blood vessels, increasing the risk for stroke.

---

d "Normal blood pressure is usually said to be 120/80 (systolic/diastolic) or less, measured in millimeters of mercury (abbreviated as mm Hg) ... The higher (systolic) number represents the pressure while the heart is beating. The lower (diastolic) number represents the pressure when the heart is resting between beats. The systolic pressure is always stated first and the diastolic pressure second." "Translating Blood Pressure Numbers." http://www.new-fitness.com/Blood_Pressure/numbers.html. Accessed October 30, 2010.

Mr. Tencion said, "I went to my family doctor yesterday and he found that my blood pressure is now 186/98. I remembered your caution not to use triptan for migraine relief if my blood pressure was elevated, so that's why I wanted to see you right away. Is there anything I can do naturally, without medication, to normalize my blood pressure so that I can continue to use triptan safely to prevent my disabling migraines?"

I nodded. "There are several natural strategies to normalize your blood pressure without the use of medications."

NATURAL WAYS TO LOWER BLOOD PRESSURE

- **Eat a diet high in fruits and vegetables.** The Dietary Approaches to Stop Hypertension (DASH) research showed that a diet that emphasizes fruits, vegetables, low-fat dairy products, less cholesterol, little refined carbohydrate and reduced-salt meals significantly lowers blood pressure to a level similar to that obtained by drug treatment within two weeks of starting the plan. DASH stresses a diet rich in fruits, vegetables, low fat, whole grains, lean meats, fish, poultry, nuts and beans. A complete description of the DASH diet developed by the U.S. National Institute of Health to lower blood pressure without medication is detailed in *The DASH Diet Action Plan*.[104]

- **Maintain body weight within 15% of ideal.** Weight reduction of as little as 10 lbs reduces blood pressure in those who are overweight. A 1986 study published in the *Journal of the Royal College of General Practitioners* showed that obese, hypertensive subjects on a weight-reducing diet who lost an average of 12 kilograms of body mass sustained over one year had a decrease in systolic pressure of 21 mmHg and in diastolic pressure of 13 mmHg.[105] The Framingham study added support to the effectiveness of an ideal weight in treatment of hypertension, showing that a weight loss of 15 lbs or more was associated with a 21% to 29% reduction in the long-term risk of hypertension.[106]

• **Limit alcohol intake to one to two ounces a day.** Studies show that consumption of more than three to four ounces of alcohol daily causes a significant, though small, elevation in blood pressure but that a lower alcohol intake of between one to two ounces a day helps maintain lower pressure in moderate drinkers compared to abstainers. The 2005 Canadian Hypertension Education Program recommends equal to or less than seven to nine drinks per week for women, and equal to or less than 14 drinks per week for men.

• **Stay active physically.**
   ◦ Studies find that just 30 minutes of moderate intensity exercise three times weekly is enough to reduce blood pressure by five to 10 mm within five weeks.[107] Walking, biking and working in the yard are just a few examples of activities that can produce an adequate workout. Thirty to 45 minutes of brisk walking at least three days a week (preferably outdoors in the fresh air, but which, during inclement weather and in winter, may be completed indoors) is more than enough exercise to normalize your blood pressure.

○ Dr. Maureen Macdonald, assistant professor of kinesiology and her co-investigators at McMaster University in Hamilton reported that simple hand-gripping exercises for a total of four minutes per hand, three times a week significantly lowers blood pressure of hypertensive patients who are already being treated with an antihypertensive medication. Dancing is an excellent exercise that combines the health enhancement benefits of music, social relationship and muscular co-ordination. Remember that life is perpetual action. All living creatures act. Death is motionless.[108]

- **Laugh down high blood pressure.** Laughter is among the best medicines for hypertension. Laughter likely improves hypertension by reducing the release of stress-related hormones such *adrenaline* and *cortisol*, resulting in a state of relaxation. Dr. Michael Miller and fellow researchers at the University of Maryland School of Medicine in Baltimore conducted a study of 20 healthy male and female volunteers who were shown funny and disturbing movies. They found that blood flow increased 22% in the test subjects during laughter and decreased by 35% when they were under stress, confirming for the first time that laughter improves circulation. Other experiments show a reduction of 10-20 mm of blood pressure in subjects after 10-30 minutes of mirthful laughter. Some studies show that 100 laughs a day provide health benefits equal to 10 minutes of aerobic exercise, such as jogging.[109]

- **Reduce salt.**
  - *The Yellow Emperor's Classic of Internal Medicine*, the ancient Chinese medical text written more than 2,000 years ago that is the main foundation for Traditional Chinese Medicine, recognized even then that too much salt causes high blood pressure and contributes to stroke. More than two millennia later, we are still consuming excessive amounts of salt and wrestling with its side effect of hypertension.

  - Canadians consume an average of 7,700 mg salt (about three teaspoons) daily. A typical North American adult eats an average of 2.5 teaspoons or 5,000 mg of salt per day. The recommended upper limit of daily salt intake for Canadians is 5.8 grams, which is equal to one teaspoon of salt and contains 2,300 mg of sodium.[110]

  - Salt is essential for regulating the fluid balance in our bodies, but like everything else, too much of it can cause health problems—particularly high blood pressure.

  - Table salt is a dietary mineral composed of 40% sodium and 60% chloride. Sea salt is obtained by the evaporation of sea water. **Sodium** is the villain in hypertension, and sodium instead of salt is usually used as unit of measurement on food labels and the Recommended Dietary Intakes for Canada. To convert the amount of sodium to its equivalent weight of salt, simply multiply the weight of sodium by 2.5. For example, if the food label states that the amount of sodium per serving is 400 mg and you want to know the corresponding quantity in terms of salt, then 400 x 2.5 = 1,000 mg of salt. To change salt to its sodium equivalent, divide the amount of salt by 2.5. For instance, if the weight of salt is 1,000 mg and you want to know how much of that is sodium, 1,000 / 2.5 = 400 mg of sodium.

The Cochrane Collaboration, a group of over 10,000 volunteers in more than 90 countries who systematically review the effects of health care interventions tested in biomedical randomized controlled trials and published the results as "Cochrane Reviews," indicates that a reduction in the average dietary sodium intake by 1,800 mg/day from 3,500 mg to 1,700 mg in Canada would result in:

- one million fewer hypertensive Canadians
- a doubling of the health care system's ability to treat high blood pressure and its control rate
- a cost savings of $430 to $538 million per year.

Data from the Cochrane Review also indicates a 5 mmHg systolic and a 2.7 mmHg diastolic reduction in blood pressure in hypertensive patients who reduced their daily dietary sodium by 1,800 mg from the customary 2,800 to 4,400 mg per day to between 1,300 mg and 2,875 mg a day.[111]

A meta-analysis of 13 studies involving 177,025 participants followed for 3.5-19 years on the relationship between the amount of habitual salt intake and stroke or total cardiovascular disease events estimated:

- that lowering daily salt intake from more than 6-12 grams to the internationally recommended less than 6 grams a day would result in reducing systolic blood pressure between 4-7 mmHg

- and, what is even more impressive, found that a reduction of 5 grams a day in regular salt intake would result in a 23% reduction in the rate of stroke and prevent 1.25 million stroke-related deaths annually worldwide.

Other investigations show that eating an extra teaspoon of salt a day increases a person's risk of stroke by 23%, but reducing salt intake by just one teaspoonful daily decreases the blood pressure of North American adults enough to lessen the stroke rate by 11%.

It is estimated that reducing sodium intake to optimal levels could lead to a 24% reduction in deaths from stroke worldwide.[112]

Another study estimates that high sodium intake kills 30 Canadians every day.[113] The Canadian Hypertension Education Program (CHEP) therefore recommends:

- reducing sodium intake to less than 2,300 mg (one teaspoon of salt) per day for people with normal blood pressure to prevent hypertension

- limiting sodium intake to between 1,500-2,300 mg (between half to one teaspoon of salt) per day in hypertensive patients

- restricting daily salt intake to less than one teaspoon. But it is not enough to simply throw away the salt shaker because the sodium in our diet comes from multiple sources, including:

○ 11% added in cooking and at the table
○ 12% occurring naturally in fresh foods we eat and water we drink
○ 77% from processed and restaurant foods.

After telling Harper Tencion these things, I then advised him that to reduce sodium intake, he must:

- stop using table salt

- avoid prepared foods since a huge amount of salt is "hidden" in processed or prepared foods

- recognize that a sodium serving of 400 mg or more is high, one of 200-400 mg per portion is moderate and 0-200 mg per helping is low

- select prepared foods with no or low sodium content per serving

- analyze the Nutrition Facts Table on the food labels carefully, finding the milligrams (mg) and *Percentage of Daily Value* for sodium

- consider that the Percentage of Daily Value refers to the amount of sodium in **one** serving of the food compared to the maximum amount of sodium we should eat a day

- choose the items with the least milligrams of sodium and the lowest Percentage of Daily Value per serving when deciding between similar products

- not eat snacks such as potato chips, pretzels or microwave popcorn

- avoid restaurant meals, particularly those from fast food chains. If you must eat in restaurants, ask the chef not to add any salt to your food

- shun salt substitutes such as *potassium chloride* or *potassium lactate* that taste salty but may cause dangerously high blood levels of potassium, especially in people with kidney disease, heart failure and in those taking diuretics such as *amiloride* and *triamterene,* as well as antihypertensive drugs, including *angiotensin-converting enzyme* (ACE) *inhibitors* and *spironolactone.*

"But how much salt is too much?" Mr. Tencion wanted to know. "Well," I said, "according to the FDA:
- 0.6 grams of sodium per 100 grams of food is a lot
- 0.1 grams of sodium per 100 grams of food is a little."

Then I reminded him:

- On food labels, the salt content is often given in grams of sodium. To convert sodium to grams of salt, multiply the quantity of sodium by 2.5. The daily limit is about 2.5 grams of sodium.

- that the amount stated on the label is often listed per 100 grams, not for the entire product. A standard ready-made meal weighs about 500 grams, so at 0.5 grams sodium per 100 grams it would contain 2.5 grams of sodium—your total recommended daily intake.

NATURAL WAYS TO REDUCE SALT INTAKE

- eat only home-cooked meals and refrain from eating in restaurants.

- limit the amount of salt in home-cooking.

- do not add salt to meals at the table.

- use a mixture of herbs and spices to flavour foods. Well-known herbal concoctions include:

  - **curry powder**, adjusted to taste using any or all of the following spices in varying amounts: coriander, turmeric, cumin, fenugreek, ginger, garlic, fennel seed, cinnamon, cloves, mustard seed, green cardamom, black cardamom, mace, nutmeg, red pepper, long pepper and black pepper

  - **five-spice powder**, commonly used in Chinese cuisine, a mixture of five spices including "Chinese cinnamon" (also known as *rougui*, the ground bark of the cassia tree, and a close relative of true cinnamon), powdered cassia buds, powdered star anise and anise seed, ginger root, and ground cloves

- choose prepared foods that contain 0.1 grams of sodium or less per 100 grams—three-quarters of the salt we eat comes from the prepackaged foods we buy.[114]

- switching everyday foods to low-sodium/reduced salt options—this means breakfast cereals, soups, biscuits, tinned vegetables and ready-made meals.

- limiting salty foods such as potato chips, salted nuts, bacon, cheese, pickles and smoked fish.

Six months later, Mr. Tencion was happy; his blood pressure was down to normal levels, and he had resumed taking his trip-tan migraine medications without fear of negative consequences.

My remembrance of Mr. Harper Tencion's consultation was interrupted by, "TRAUMA ALERT, 15 MINUTES. TRAUMA ALERT, 15 MINUTES."

Lower Your Blood Pressure

- Consume no more than five grams of salt (one teaspoon) which is equivalent to approximately two grams of sodium a day
- Eat home-cooked low salt foods
- Use herbs and spices to flavour your home-cooked meals.

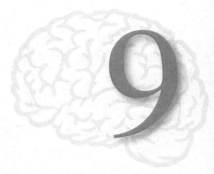

diet defeats diabetes

"Let food be thy medicine and medicine be thy food."

~ HIPPOCRATES

"TRAUMA ALERT, 15 MINUTES. TRAUMA ALERT, 15 MINUTES," barked the hospital public address loudspeakers. Time speeding away irretrievably concentrated my attention on the stroke crisis in front of me.

I glanced at the continuous blood pressure monitor firmly attached to Mr. Patience's paralyzed left arm. 196/98. *Still too high to administer tPA safely.*

"Are his blood tests back yet?" was my urgent question to stroke nurse Florence.

"Right here, Dr. Veloso. All his blood parameters are within normal limits—except for *glucose*, which is markedly elevated." she answered.

"My husband is diabetic but hasn't been taking his medication as prescribed because of his fear of side effects,"[a] Mrs. Patience said. She'd obviously heard Nurse Florence's pronounce-

a These side effects of diabetes medications include low blood sugar, upset stomach, skin rash, weight gain, weakness, tiredness, dizziness, shortness of breath, nausea, diarrhea, liver toxicity, anemia, heart attack, edema with heart failure and headache ment that her husband's blood sugar was dangerously high. "Are there any natural remedies he could have tried?"

A new study has found that the number of Canadians with *diabetes mellitus* will jump from the current 2.5 million to 3.7 million over the next 10 years. In other words, there are 20 newly diagnosed Canadian diabetics every hour and one new diabetic will be identified every 90 seconds for the next several decades. The cost of diabetes to the Canadian economy will climb from $12.2 billion today to $16.9 billion over the next decade, the report says.[115] The reasons for the prevalence of diabetes are:

- Canada's changing ethnicities, understanding that certain races are more susceptible to the disease
- The increasingly aging Canadian population—the risk of diabetes increases with age
- Our expanding obesity problem
- General inactivity
- Canada's unhealthy dietary habits.

Most people today understand that **diabetes mellitus** is a disease that affects the body's ability to secrete *insulin* and/or to utilize it efficiently. It is important to remember that there are two types of diabetes mellitus for a better understanding of the most favorable management strategies to control the disease.

Type 1 diabetes, also known as i*nsulin-dependent diabetes mellitus* (IDDM) or *juvenile diabetes*, is caused by a lack of insulin secretion from the beta cells of a pancreas usually damaged by viral infection or autoimmune disease—although heredity sometimes contributes to the injury. Type 1 diabetes is therefore a disease of insulin *deficiency* and is best treated with insulin injections, since the hormone is inactivated by digestive enzymes if taken orally.

Type 2 diabetes, also called *non-insulin dependent diabetes mellitus* (NIDDM) or *adult onset diabetes*, is due to the body's reduced response to the effects of insulin. Type 2 diabetes is therefore an illness of insulin *resistance*. Type 2 diabetes accounts for between 80 to 90% of all known cases of diabetes, and, as its name implies, affects mostly adults aged 50 or older. Type 2 diabetes is usually associated with obesity, although the relationship is yet poorly understood, but some studies suggest that there are fewer insulin receptors in obese people compared to lean people.[116] Type 2 diabetes can be treated with medications that increase insulin sensitivity or stimulate the pancreas to produce more insulin.

If not managed properly, Type 2 diabetes may deteriorate to the Type 1 form, in which case insulin injections will be needed to keep blood sugar levels in the normal range. Both types of diabetes mellitus—but particularly Type 2—can be improved by weight loss and exercise. In fact, there's a lot of evidence that natural strategies are effective in the prevention and improvement of diabetes. Those who have diabetes have a stroke risk two to three times greater than those who do not.

I told Mrs. Patience that:

- a study from Finland showed that changing eating and exercise habits can definitely prevent the onset of diabetes in people at high risk for the disease. The Finnish Diabetes Prevention Study of 523 adults with impaired glucose tolerance confirmed that a low-calorie, low-fat and high-fibre diet plus moderate-intensity physical activity of at least 150 minutes per week that reduced approximately 5% of the subject's initial body weight can decrease the risk of developing diabetes by more than 50% after four years.[117]

- The European Prospective Investigation of Cancer–Norfolk Prospective Study conducted by Dr. Anne-Helen Harding and associates in 2008 concluded that high *Vitamin C*, fruit and vegetables prevent diabetes.[118]

- The Intake of Fruit, Vegetables and Fruit Juices, and Risk of Diabetes in Women survey of 71,346 non-diabetic female nurses followed for 18 years by Dr. Lydia A. Bazzano from Tulane University School of Public Health and Tropical Medicine in New Orleans, Louisiana concluded that consumption of green leafy vegetables and fruit (not juices) was associated with a lower risk of diabetes among women.[119]

- An analysis of data on 83,818 female nurses followed over 16 years by researchers at the Harvard School of Public Health in Boston reported that those who ate an ounce of nuts or a tablespoon of peanut butter at least five times a week reduced their risk of developing Type 2 diabetes by 20% compared to those who rarely or never ate nuts.[120]

- Moreover, a study conducted by Dr. Julie R. Palmer at Boston University of 43,960 African Americans followed over 10 years found that consuming one to two regular soft drinks, fruit drinks or fruit juice (excluding grapefruit and orange) was associated with a 24% to 31% increased risk of developing Type 2 diabetes. The researchers indicated that weight gain from consumption of the sugary drinks was the culprit responsible for the increased risk.[121]

- Even more compelling was the analysis of 41 trials involving a total of 1,674 diabetics and non-diabetics by researchers at St. Michael's Hospital in

Toronto, which substantiated that eating legumes either alone or added to a high-fibre diet lowered fasting glucose levels in people with Type 2 diabetes to those attained by oral diabetic medications.[122]

I told Mrs. Patience about the **Glycemic Index (GI)** developed by Dr. David J. Jenkins and colleagues at the University of Toronto. The GI is a measurement of the effects of carbohydrate-rich foods on blood sugar levels that directly impacts diabetes and obesity control. The GI categorizes carbohydrate-containing foods into three general classes:

- **High Glycemic Index Foods**
  which cause a fast rise in blood-glucose levels

- **Intermediate Glycemic Index Foods**
  which produce a moderate rise in blood-glucose

- **Low Glycemic Index Foods**
  which cause a slower rise in blood-sugar.

EATING LOW GI FOODS ...

- controls blood glucose level
- improves cholesterol profile
- curbs appetite
- reduces risk of heart attack
- lowers danger of developing diabetes[123]

Diabetics and pre-diabetic individuals should consider GI when planning their meals. Highly refined foods such as white sugar or flour generally have a high glycemic index, whereas unprocessed produce—including high-fibre whole grains, vegetables, fruits, legumes, nuts, pulses and seeds—have a lower glycemic index and may prevent or even *reverse* diabetes mellitus. Diabetics and pre-diabetics should practise these principles of healthy eating:

- Eat three preferably home-cooked meals daily
- Avoid high Glycemic Index foods
- Reduce the amount of fat (especially saturated) in their diet
- Consume generous servings of fruits, vegetables and nuts every day
- Minimize highly refined foods
- Consult your physician and/or dietician regularly

"And there's similar proof that exercise is therapeutic for diabetics!" I told Mrs. Patience. Indeed, many studies show that 20 to 30 minutes of moderate intensity exercise three times a week not only *prevents* but also *improves* Type 2 diabetes:

- the Diabetes Prevention Program Research Group reported in the *New England Journal of Medicine* their comparative study of 3,234 high risk diabetics. They randomly assigned one-third of the study participants to taking a placebo, another third to taking the oral diabetic medication *metformin*, and the remaining third to intensive lifestyle intervention, consisting of 150 minutes of moderate intensity physical activity (mostly brisk walking) per week, plus adherence to a low-fat, low-calorie diet to achieve a weight reduction of at least 7% of their initial body weight. The study showed that the incidence of diabetes was reduced by 58% in the lifestyle intervention group and by 31% with the metformin-treated participants compared to the group taking a placebo, proving that exercise in combination with healthy diet is more effective than medication in the prevention of diabetes mellitus.[124]

- Another study titled "Effects of diet and exercise in preventing NIDDM in people with impaired glucose tolerance. The Da Qing IGT and Diabetes Study" conducted by Dr. X. R. Pan and colleagues from the Department of Endocrinology, China-Japan Friendship Hospital, Beijing found that exercise with or without dietary discretion in 577 high risk diabetic subjects resulted in up to a 46% reduction in their risk of developing diabetes.[125]

"There are many scientific studies published in medical journals confirming that moderate intensity exercises of approximately 30 minutes three times weekly can lower the risk of Type 2 diabetes by up to 60%," I informed Mrs. Patience.

Some of the precautions *all* diabetics, but particularly those who suffer from Type 1, must observe before engaging in exercises are:

- Having a medical check-up prior to and periodically throughout the exercise program
- Monitoring blood sugar levels carefully before, during, and after workouts and adjusting insulin dosages accordingly
- Avoiding exercise if glucose levels are higher than 300 mg or lower than 100 mg per 100 ml
- Drinking plenty of fluids
- Avoiding strenuous physical activities that may damage delicate blood vessels in the eye already at risk from diabetes for retinopathy and loss of vision.

"TRAUMA ALERT, 12 MINUTES," broadcast the hospital's public address system as soon as I finished talking about the natural methods of alleviating and preventing diabetes. I needed to assess Prudence Patience's husband once more.

"Quick! What's Mr. Patience's blood pressure now?" I asked, glancing up at the monitor.

Diet Defeats Diabetes

- Stick to a healthy, low-calorie, low-fat, low-glycemic index, high-fibre diet
- Participate in 30 minutes of moderate intensity exercises three times a week.

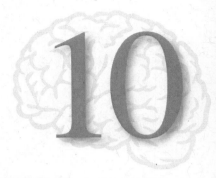

cholesterol cleansing clears circulation

"The rest of the world lives to eat, while I eat to live."

~ SOCRATES

"190/98," Nurse Florence answered calmly.

I checked the continuous blood pressure monitor wrapped snugly around Mr. Patience paralyzed left arm and stared at the monitor to verify that his blood pressure was still dangerously elevated. Only 12 minutes remaining before the window slammed shut for the safe administration of brain-saving tPA.

"Is there anything more we can do to lower his blood pressure before our time's up?" I implored Dr. Critico.

"Yes," Dr. Critico stated confidently as he administered another bolus of 80 mg of labetalol intravenously to Mr. Patience. "It may take five minutes or so before his blood pressure lowers to a safer level," the intensivist said, his voice optimistic.

While waiting for Mr. Patience's blood pressure to cooperate, I elicited more pertinent medical history about our patient by asking his wife if she knew of anything else that might have contributed to her husband's stroke.

"Well," Prudence Patience said, "Victor does have high cholesterol."

High cholesterol, hypertension, diabetes and smoking are generally known as "the four horsemen of apoplexy" and Victor Patience had been prescribed several cholesterol-lowering drugs:

- **Statins** lower the production of cholesterol in the liver by blocking an enzyme called *hydroxy-methylglutaryl-coenzyme A reductase* (HMG-CoA reductase). These lipid-lowering drugs are referred to as *HMG-CoA reductase inhibitors.*

- **Resins** (also called *bile acid sequestrants*) bind during digestion to aid bile acids made by the liver using cholesterol and prompt the body to eliminate the combination, which in turn uses the excess cholesterol to make more bile acids, resulting in a lowering of overall blood cholesterol levels.

- **Cholesterol absorption inhibitors** lower cholesterol by reducing the intestinal absorption of the lipid, although recent studies show that this type of antihyperlipidemic drug may actually worsen atherosclerosis, resulting in a higher incidence of heart disease. A new head-to-head trial has revealed that the much-less-expensive *extended-released niacin* is superior to cholesterol absorption inhibitors.[126]

- **Fibrates** (also called *fibric acid derivatives*) lower bodily lipids by reducing the amount of triglycerides mainly via stimulation of the enzymatic activity of *lipase,* resulting in better clearance of circulating triglyceride-rich lipoproteins.[a]

- *Niacin* (also called *nicotinic acid*) is a B vitamin that, in large doses, lowers triglycerides by preventing the compounding of enzymes that results in their creation. Niacin also increases high density lipoprotein cholesterol (HDL) by preventing liver cells from accumulating the good cholesterol. The good cholesterol is therefore free to circulate in the blood to do its good work instead of being held in the liver not doing anything (like money stored under the mattress at home instead of being circulated to improve the economy).

Unfortunately, Mr. Patience didn't always take these medications regularly, his wife told me, because of the actual or feared side effects of the drugs, including:

- Muscle aches and/or weakness from *statin myopathy* and the more serious *rhabdomyolysis* that may lead to *renal failure* [b]
- Liver damage
- Diarrhea or constipation
- Abdominal pain, cramps, bloating or gas
- Nausea
- Vomiting
- Headache

---

a Lipase is an enzyme secreted in the digestive tract that motivates the breakdown of large fat molecules (triglycerides) into individual fatty acids that can then be absorbed into the bloodstream. Lipoproteins are the protein and fat molecules that carry cholesterol.

b "Statin myopathy is an inflammation of the muscles caused by a statin medication. The most severe form of statin myopathy causes destruction of the muscle tissue, which is called **rhabdomyolysis** ... The most common symptoms of statin myopathy include muscle pain and muscle weakness. Additional symptoms of worsening statin myopathy include muscle swelling, and pink, red, or brown urine ... Treatment for severe rhabdomyolysis may include kidney dialysis." http://www.freemd.com/statin-myopathy/. Accessed November 3, 2010.

- ○ Drowsiness
- ○ Dizziness
- ○ Rash
- ○ Sleep problems
- ○ Interaction with other medications, even grapefruit, due to interference with the liver enzyme CYP 3A4, resulting in an elevation of statins, possibly to toxic levels
- ○ Possible triggering of ALS (Lou Gehrig's disease).

Cholesterol is a natural fatty substance critical to the body's needs for the production of several essential hormones, including *testosterone, estrogen, dihydroepiandrosterone, progesterone* and *cortisol,* as well as for the synthesis of *bile acids,* which is necessary for the absorption of fats, and *Vitamin D* now known to be a protection against cancer, and which decreases the incidence of auto-immune diseases such as rheumatoid arthritis and prevents osteoporosis.

Cholesterol is also a crucial component of cell membranes, particularly of neurons, where it contributes to the physiological transmission of nerve impulses. The liver normally produces our daily requirement of about 1,000 milligrams of cholesterol. But our daily cholesterol production often has a surplus, coming mostly from the fatty meats and dairy products in our diet.

Cholesterol is naturally a greasy, relatively insoluble fatty compound. To improve its solubility and mobility, cholesterol combines with certain proteins to form *lipoproteins*, which are more dissolvable in blood and therefore easier to transport in the bloodstream.

There are several types of lipoproteins but the most abundant are **low-density lipoproteins (LDL)**, whose main function is to transport cholesterol from the liver to tissue cells and **high-density lipoprotein (HDL),** which carries old or used cholesterol to the liver for recycling or elimination.

Currently, it is the generally accepted medical opinion that elevated blood cholesterol, particularly the low-density lipoprotein cholesterol (so called "bad" cholesterol) causes *atherosclerosis* (hardening of the arteries), leading to stroke and heart attack, while high levels of high-density lipoprotein cholesterol (so called "good" cholesterol) protects against cardiovascular disease by removing the cholesterol deposited in atherosclerotic plaques, thereby preventing strokes and heart attacks.

Is there proof that cholesterol, a natural substance crucial to the integrity of the body's cellular structure and function, is—at the same time—harmful to the cardiovascular system?

Not much. More than a century ago, investigators found that rabbits force-fed a cholesterol-rich diet developed lesions in their arterial walls that were notably similar to human atherosclerotic damage. Other investigators then jumped onto the high-cholesterol diet = atherosclerosis bandwagon even as the original researchers cautioned that *hypercholesterolemia* (a high cholesterol level) was probably only one of several triggers for the disease, although perhaps a major co-conspirator. Subsequent investigation revealed that it was the oxidized form of ("bad") low-density lipoprotein cholesterol (naturally occurring standard low-density lipoprotein that has been oxidized by free radicals) that is the principal instigator of atherosclerosis.

This "lipid hypothesis" was consequently revised to conform to the more scientifically accurate concept that the elevation of oxidized, "bad" low-density lipoprotein cholesterol—and not high blood cholesterol levels—is the true culprit behind atherosclerosis. However, emerging research indicates that even *this* belief of an elevated oxidized "bad" low-density-lipoprotein-cholesterol-causing-atherosclerosis scenario might be overly simplistic.

Recent investigations reveal that atherosclerosis has multiple causes and that there are several other major triggers of atherosclerosis. The cause most to blame for atherosclerosis appears to be inflammation of any sort, but particularly those from infections. The same studies found that statins reduce cardiovascular disease not by lowering cholesterol but by decreasing *C-reactive protein,* which is a very sensitive marker of inflammation.[127]

Current research has revealed that statins reduce deaths due to heart disease but not the stroke rate. With little change in blood cholesterol levels but a significant reduction of inflammatory markers such as C-reactive protein, studies indicate that the benefits of statins are likely due to their anti-inflammatory properties rather than to their well-publicized anti-cholesterol action.

Scientific research has also found that statins benefit only a select group of middle-aged males with pre-existing coronary heart disease. The Prospective Study of Pravastatin in the Elderly at Risk (PROSPER study) did find that a statin reduced incidents of death due to heart disease, but the benefit was neutralized by an equal number of cancer deaths. The same research failed to show any positive effect of the statin on stroke prevention. Studies with another statin showed that the cholesterol-lowering medications might be associated with an increase in all-cause mortality in healthy hypercholesterolemic individuals.[128] This means that the number of deaths of all kinds is increased by cholesterol-lowering medications; otherwise healthy hypercholesterolemic individuals who use statins might have a higher chance of dying from any disease and not just heart disease or stroke.

The conclusion of a recently completed trial titled "Justification for the Use of Statins in Prevention: an Intervention Trial Evaluating Rosuvastatin (JUPITER)" was that a particular statin significantly reduced major cardiovascular events in healthy people with elevated inflammatory C-reactive protein markers but without hyperlipidemia. However, this again validates inflammation and not hypercholesterolemia as the principal cause of atherosclerosis.[129]

A new study of 6,113 adults participants divided into five

groups based on their intake of sugar in the National Health and Nutrition Examination Survey from 1999 to 2006 found that subjects in the highest sugar-consuming group had about a three times higher risk of having lower "good" HDL cholesterol than the lowest consuming group, whereas those in the middle sugar-intake group had a one and a half times greater risk of having low HDL levels than those in the lowest consumption group. The study found that those who consumed food with higher levels of sugar showed a risk ranging from 50% to 300% higher of reduced levels of "good" HDL cholesterol.[130]

Other research shows that the reduction in death rates due to statins are no greater than, and often inferior to, lifestyle changes such as regular exercise, smoking cessation, weight loss, stress reduction, sleep sufficiency, liberal eating of a vegetable- and fruit-rich diet, avoidance of added sugar in prepared foods and drinks, plus supplementing with omega-3 fatty acids.

"Still," I told Mrs. Patience, "*nobody should reduce or stop taking cholesterol-lowering medication on the basis of these clarifications.* Hopefully, people will choose to add to their cholesterol-lowering regime with healthy lifestyle choices."

I hoped she understood that inflammation is probably guiltier than high cholesterol of causing strokes and that infection is the most common trigger of inflammation. Further, lifestyle changes can reduce inflammation even better than—and without the side effects of—statins.

There are several natural lifestyle modifications that lower the risk of inflammation and are equal to or better than widely prescribed cholesterol-lowering drugs.

NATURAL WAYS TO LOWER CHOLESTEROL

- Regular exercise
- Eating small, oily fish twice a week or two capsules of 500 mg omega-3 fatty acid daily
- Achieving and maintaining ideal body weight
- Eating a diet rich in fibre, fruits, vegetables, whole grains, lean white meats—and one low in sugar, salt, trans or saturated fats
- Good dental hygiene with daily teeth flossing.

"Good dental hygiene!?" she exclaimed. "Do you think that my husband's gum disease could have contributed to his stroke?" asked an astonished Mrs. Patience.

A Healthy Lifestyle Lowers Cholesterol

Supplement your cholesterol-lowering regime with a healthy lifestyle by:

- exercising regulary
- not smoking
- maintaining an ideal weight
- reducing stress
- sleeping well
- eating a vegetable- and fruit-rich diet
- supplementing with omega-3 fatty acids
- not reducing or stopping cholesterol-lowering drugs without consulting your physician.

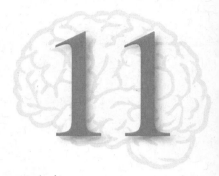

11

preventing periodontitis prevents strokes

"Up and down and round and round
I brush my teeth to keep them sound.
To keep them sound and clean and white
I brush them morning, noon and night."

~ Anonymous

"Trauma alert. Ten minutes," blurted the loudspeakers again. Only ten minutes left to save Mr. Patience from his disabling stroke and his blood pressure was still too high.

"188/96," the stroke nurse told me as I checked the monitor.

"How are you doing?" I asked Mr. Patience.

"I still can't move my left side," he slurred. "When are you going to make me better?"

"Soon, very soon," I told him as I wiped the saliva drooling down the left side of his mouth.

"Where is his wife?" I asked Florence after noticing that Mrs. Patience was no longer beside the stroke victim's stretcher.

"She rushed out of the room—something about having to cancel a dental appointment," Florence said.

Mrs. Patience returned to her husband's bedside, explaining

that she had left to phone the dentist to cancel Victor's appointment for a gum disease evaluation that was to have taken place that morning.

"But you haven't yet told me how gum disease could have caused my husband's stroke."

In 1990, I was wine-tasting on a Panama Canal cruise. While the sommelier praised the qualities of a Niagara Shiraz, I was busy touting the health benefits, particularly that of stroke prevention, of red wine to fellow oenophiles seated around my table.

"If you're really interested in learning something new about stroke prevention, then come to the seminar I'm presenting tomorrow morning regarding the relationship of periodontitis to stroke," said the distinguished silver-haired gentleman seated beside me. Though I suspected this was his way of telling me to be quiet so he could hear what the sommelier was saying, I was nevertheless intrigued. I thought I knew all the major modifiable risk factors of stroke prevention: smoking, diabetes, hypertension, physical inactivity, hypercholesterolemia and obesity, as well the unmodifiable causes such as heredity, history of stroke, ethnicity and gender. But gum disease?

When the sommelier had moved to the next table, I turned and introduced myself, saying in addition, "Sorry if I distracted you. As you've probably guessed, I'm a neurologist."

"Pleased to meet you. I'm Dr. Denton Flostine and, as *you* might have guessed, I'm a dentist. There's no need to apologize. And I sincerely hope you will listen to my talk on the relationship between periodontitis and stroke tomorrow morning at 9," said the gracious dentist.

Even though I'd skipped my morning jog, I was still five minutes late to listen to Dr. Flostine's seminar. I quietly entered the lecture theatre and sat down in the nearest empty chair. An estimated 50 attendees—presumably all dentists—were already assembled and Dr. Flostine had begun to present a compelling case implicating periodontitis as a principal villain responsible for the second highest cause of mortality in Canada.

"*Inflammation*," Dr. Flostine said, "was recognized 150 years ago as a cause of atherosclerosis by Dr. Rudolf Virchow, the father of modern pathology. Over the past century, scientific proof has accumulated, confirming that inflammation is likely the final common pathway of all the risk factors of stroke and heart attack.

"What is **inflammation?**" he continued. "It is the cellular response to tissue injury. An increase of C-reactive protein (CRP)—diagnosed through a *high sensitivity C-reactive blood test (hs-CRP)*—is the hallmark of inflammation. Elevated CRP in the blood is commonly seen in infections (whether viral or bacterial), malignancies and auto-immune diseases but also may be due to other, seemingly non-inflammatory conditions such as obesity, diabetes mellitus, *uremia,*[a] hypertension, marked physical exertion, oral hormone replacement therapy, sleep disturbances, chronic fatigue, alcoholism, physical inactivity and even depression."

I learned a lot from Dr. Flostine. Until recently, gum disease was probably the most common yet unrecognized cause of the elevation of C-reactive protein. One of the main triggers of inflammation is infection. The notion that infection can cause atherosclerosis by way of inflammation and end in stroke and heart attack is also not new. A century and a half ago, the father of modern medicine, Sir William Osler, acknowledged infection as one of the principal factors of atherosclerosis.[131]

In the first half of the 20th century, scientists were attracted to the more topical and glamorous risk factors of hypertension, smoking and hypercholesterolemia, resulting in the neglect of infection as a cause of stroke. The hypothesis of infections causing atherosclerosis was revived in the early 1980s by Dr. Barry Marshall and Dr. Robin Warren, who discovered that peptic ulcer, long believed to be triggered by stress, and its resulting

---

a The illness accompanying kidney failure.

stomach hyperacidity was in fact caused by a bacterium named *Helicobacter pylori (H. pylori).*[132]

What a wake-up call to researchers! If microbes can cause stomach and duodenal ulcers, why not atherosclerosis? Extensive investigations by dedicated researchers over the past five decades show that the four risk factors of hypertension, diabetes, smoking and hypercholesterolemia account for—at most—60% of strokes. But Yasunori Sawayamaa and his associates from Japan investigating the relationship between *H. pylori* infection and acute ischemic stroke in 62 first-stroke patients and 143 controls learned that *H. pylori* infection is associated with an increased risk of ischemic stroke.[133]

The hunt for microscopic organisms causing disabling strokes has intensified since. Numerous studies over the past 30 years have revealed a close association between germs—notably *Chlamydia pneumoniae, cytomegalovirus, herpes simplex virus* and *H. pylori*—and stroke. Investigations have shown that infections can trigger atherosclerosis by damaging the lining of blood vessels, leading to the activation of the inflammatory process, including deposits of cholesterol in the injured artery. The link between microorganisms and stroke is particularly strong in chronic infections with persistent inflammation.

The most common but generally overlooked chronic infection is gum disease. **Gingivitis** or **periodontitis** is an inflammation of the gums due to plaque, a film of bacteria and food particles deposited on the surfaces of teeth. Gingivitis is conservatively estimated to affect at least 50% of adults, making gum disease probably the most common source of inflammation and therefore a major cause of stroke.[134] There is considerable evidence supporting the role of gum disease as a cause of stroke:

- A study by K. J. Mattila and associates from the First Department of Medicine of Helsinki University Central Hospital found that dental health was significantly worse in patients with acute myocardial infarction than in controls.[135]

- Research by Lorelei A. Mucci and colleagues from the Department of Epidemiology, Harvard School of Public Health of 15,273 Swedish twins followed for 37 years revealed that oral disease was associated with excess cardiovascular disease risk, independent of genetic factors.[136]

- Investigations by Yukihito Higashi and co-researchers from Hiroshima, Japan discovered that periodontitis is associated with *endothelial dysfunction*[b] in subjects without cardiovascular risk factors and in hypertensive subjects.[137]

- Pirkko J. Pussinen and fellow examiners from Helsinki, Finland followed 6,051 individuals for up to 10 years and verified that exposure to periodontal pathogens or *endotoxins*[c] induces systemic inflammation, leading to an increased risk for cerebrovascular disease.[138]

- An inquiry by Axel Spahr and associates in Germany reported an association between periodontitis and the presence of coronary heart disease in 2006.[139]

- New research by C.E. Dörfer and co-investigators reported that periodontitis is an independent risk factor for stroke.[140]

---

b Deterioration of blood vessel walls.
c Toxins contained in microorganisms that are released when the microorganism is broken down or dies.

- Steven P. Engebretson and co-researchers' study reported panoramic oral radiograph evidence that severe periodontal bone loss is independently associated with carotid atherosclerosis.[141]

- Dr. Kaumudi J. Joshipura and co-workers from Harvard School of Dental Medicine studied 41,380 men between the ages of 40 to 75 and followed them for 12 years, confirming that men who loss seven or more of their normal complement of 32 teeth to periodontal disease had a 57% higher risk of stroke compared those who retained 25 teeth or more.[142]

- Dr. J.D. Beck and co-investigators from Chapel Hill, North Carolina studied 6,796 subjects aged 52 to 75 from 1996 to 1998, concluding that periodontitis was an independent risk factor for stroke in more than 8% of the participants.[143]

- Dr. Armin J. Grau and co-workers from the University of Heidelberg in Germany examined 303 patients within seven days after acute ischemic stroke or transient ischemic attack, and compared them to 300 population and 168 hospital controls with nonvascular and noninflammatory neurological diseases. They found that subjects with severe periodontitis had a 4.3% higher risk of cerebral ischemia than subjects with mild or without periodontitis, and concluded that periodontitis was an independent risk factor for stroke.[144]

- Dr. Tiejian Wu and co-investigators from the State University of New York at Buffalo examined the link between gum disease and the risk of having a stroke in nearly 10,000 adults between the ages of 25 and 75. The research, conducted from 1972-1992, found that periodontitis was a significant and independent risk factor for any cerebrovascular event and was associated with a two-fold increase in the risk for stroke.[145]

- In yet another study, Dr. S.J. Sim and associates from the School of Dentistry at the National University of Seoul, Korea compared 265 stroke patients to 214 non-stroke individuals and concluded that there is a four-fold increase risk of stroke in those with periodontitis.[146]

After he presented more than enough evidence to convict periodontitis beyond a reasonable doubt of being a co-conspirator—if not the principal instigator—of stroke, Dr. Flostine recommended the following natural ways to prevent this serious, but until recently overlooked, plague.

NATURAL WAYS TO AVOID PERIODONTITIS

- Visit the dentist once a year
- Brush teeth gently with a soft-bristled toothbrush after every meal
- Floss teeth after very meal
- Avoid eating sugar or other refined carbohydrates to prevent plaque build-up on teeth
- Maintain a balanced, healthy diet
- Boost circulation in gums by massaging them with your fingertips
- Keep your toothbrush clean of bacteria by disinfecting it, preferably with 3% hydrogen peroxide, between brushings

- Change to a new toothbrush every month
- Use a tongue scraper after brushing or flossing to prevent bacteria buildup
- Use a mixture of baking soda and hydrogen peroxide for brushing teeth to prevent gingivitis, whiten teeth and freshen breath. Add one tablespoonful of 3% hydrogen peroxide to 2 tablespoons of baking soda in a cup. Mix the two together to form a paste. Dip your toothbrush into the paste and brush as you would if you were using toothpaste. Rinse your mouth well after using the peroxide and baking soda mixture. Use the mixture only once or twice a week. More frequent brushing with abrasive baking soda can damage tooth enamel.
- Use 3% hydrogen peroxide or, if preferred, a mixture of equal amounts of 3% hydrogen peroxide and water to brush teeth and/or rinse mouth the rest of the time.
- Always brush gently with a circular motion using a soft or extra-soft tooth brush.

My memory of one of the most professional and personally rewarding continuing medical education seminars I'd been to ended abruptly with the renewed alarm: "TRAUMA ALERT, FIVE MINUTES!"

Time was quickly running out for Mr. Patience to safely receive life-saving tPA. Was his blood pressure finally low enough to begin treatment?

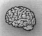 *Healthy Teeth and Gums Mean Healthy Brains*

- Brush with a soft-bristle toothbrush and floss teeth after each meal
- Use homemade dental paste of one tablespoon 3% hydrogen peroxide plus two tablespoons of baking soda to brush teeth one to two times weekly in addition to regular brushing
- Use either 3% hydrogen peroxide or a mixture of equal amounts of 3% hydrogen peroxide and water to brush teeth and/or rinse mouth the rest of the time.

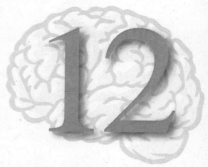

serenity stops strokes

"Man is made by his beliefs. As he believes, so he is."

~ BHAGAVAD GITA

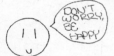

"Mr. Patience's blood pressure is now 170/100," came the swift response from Nurse Florence.

Finally! "Is his tPA ready?" I asked.

"It's standing by. We translated his weight of 230 pounds to 104.5 kilograms. The recommended dose for tPA in the treatment of acute ischemic stroke is nine milligrams per kilogram of body weight to a maximum total dose of 90 milligrams. The pharmacist prepared 90 milligrams of tPA for Mr. Patience about an hour ago," Florence confirmed.

"Quick!" I urged. "Program the intravenous infusion pump to administer a bolus of nine milligrams or 10% of the total dose of 90 milligrams of tPA over one to two minutes, and then instill the remaining 81 milligrams in a constant infusion over one hour. Also, continue to maintain his blood pressure below 175/110 by adjusting the rate of the labetalol drip," I ordered.

"Done," said Florence, and I saw the tPA start running into Mr. Patience's vein.

"How are you doing?" I asked the patient.

"Fine. Am I getting the blood clot-busting medicine now?" asked the anxious stroke victim.

"Yes," I assured him, patting his arm.

My focus on the tPA dripping into his vein was interrupted by one of the ER nurses. "Dr. Veloso, the trauma patients have arrived and Dr. Emerge wants you to take a look at one of the victims—he's unconscious and paralyzed on the left side just like Mr. Patience."

I asked Florence to continue keeping a close watch over Mr. Patience and his blood pressure before rushing to examine the accident casualty. The unresponsive man had a large bruise on the right side of his head and his right pupil was larger than the left. Experience immediately told me that he had a rapidly expanding blood clot on the right side of his head between the skull and the dural covering of the brain. It had to be evacuated without delay if his life was to be saved.

"Get him to CT, stat! And get me the neurosurgeon on-call right away," I directed the nurse.

"How did the accident happen?" I wondered aloud as the co-matose man was rapidly wheeled away by an orderly.

"The emergency medical service team said that his wife—who suffered only minor bruises—told them that the victim had a seizure that caused the accident. She believes that the convul-sion was due to a side effect of the antidepressants her husband was prescribed a week or so ago," Dr. Emerge volunteered.

"Dr. Veloso, Dr. Benjamin Kasie is on line two," the nurse called out.

"Ben, I have a patient here with an *epidural hematoma*. Please come right away," I requested the neurosurgeon over the phone.

"I'll be there in 15 minutes," Dr. Kasie promised. "Kindly no-tify the operating room to get ready."

True to his word, Dr. Kasie was in the ER less than 15 minutes later to review with me the CT scan that had just been completed. The scan confirmed the presence of a huge epidural hematoma compressing the right half of the car accident victim's brain. He was whisked to the operating room where his life was saved by the emergency removal of the epidural hematoma.

I returned to Mr. Patience's room.

"How is Mr. Patience doing?" I checked with the stroke nurse.

"Great! His vital signs are stable. His blood pressure varies between 160 to 170 systolic and 90 to 100 diastolic. He's also awake and alert. The tPA infusion has another 30 minutes to run," Florence replied.

As I left Victor Patience's room, I met Mrs. Patience coming from the other end of the hallway. She was agitated, the lines on her forehead pleated in concern, and she was talking a mile a minute. "Oh, Dr. Veloso!" she said, "I just met the accident victim's wife crying in the washroom. I couldn't help but overhear what was going on with her husband and told her how sorry I was. I told her that my husband had just a stroke too, and that he'd just started the treatment that might save his life.

"She told me that *her* husband had a seizure while driving, causing the crash and his severe head injury. She thinks the seizure was a side effect of the antidepressant he's been taking for several days. I didn't know that antidepressants could cause stroke!

"This really worries me, Dr. Veloso. Victor and I lost our life savings of mutual fund investments a little while ago—we thought our nest egg was safe but we were swindled by fraudulent fund managers whose schemes unraveled when the stock market crashed. Victor's been depressed and anxious ever since. I tried to comfort him but he's been inconsolable.

"His psychiatrist prescribed antidepressants, which not only did *not* improve his doom and gloom but instead caused intolerable side effects like weight gain, constipation, dry mouth and drowsiness. *Now* I learn that antidepressants can also cause convulsions and sometimes even strokes! Oh, I wish there were natural, non-drug remedies my husband could take to treat his emotional problems instead!" Mrs. Patience said.

Her concern triggered my memory of a meeting I'd had with a good friend several years earlier. Mr. Brelex Notable was a retired pharmacist, a very astute businessman who had made a fortune establishing a chain of retail pharmacies in the 1970s. Mr. Notable was rumoured to have retired with more than $40 million when he sold his very profitable business to an Eastern Canadian pharmaceutical company, which then expanded nationally. Like most prairie retirees, Mr. Notable had moved to the West Coast. He bought a huge mansion high on a hill facing English Bay, which was reputed to have 28 washrooms—some of which had gold-plated toilets! He had often invited other members of the "nouveau riche" to his home to discuss stock market investment strategies.

One Sunday morning about three years ago, Mr. Notable phoned, asking to talk to me. He said that he was on his way to Toronto for a meeting with his bankruptcy trustee, and that he wanted to check with me how it might affect his health.

"I lost my entire fortune in the high-tech bubble stock market crash," he'd said. "I invested half my assets in a stock the analysts claimed was the biggest-ever gold discovery, but which turned out to be the greatest-ever salting fraud in mining history! I lost the other half of my savings by entrusting it to a technology company that was a heavy hitter on the Toronto Stock Exchange—who knew they were cooking the books?! I was not only financially ruined but I felt I had lost face. I was deeply depressed. Then I recalled Henry Thoreau's words: 'simplify, simplify, simplify.'[147] I also remembered Thoreau saying that 'a man is rich in proportion to the things he can afford to do without,'[148] and Socrates' teaching that 'the secret of happiness … is not found in seeking more, but in developing the capacity to enjoy less.'

"After contemplating this for some time, I realized that the three basic essentials of life—food, shelter and clothing—were still readily available to me. And the other two necessities of air and water are naturally abundant. I was relieved to find that I still possessed all the basics necessities of life! I was also delighted to realize that I do not, in fact, *need* wealth to survive. After all, how many toilets—even of solid gold!—can I sit on at one time?

"At the same time, I recognized that there is another vital requisite to sustain life, and that is health. Life without health is not viable. Health is the only one of life's necessities that is neither transferable nor negotiable. Health is not procurable or saleable. Health is solely the owner's maintainable! No one and nothing can be tasked with the preservation of one's well-being. Health is both physical and mental. I am physically fit but emotionally ailing. I am contented but not serene. I feel anxious and depressed. And that's why I'm calling, Dr. Veloso.

"My family physician referred me to a psychiatrist who wants me to go on medication, but, as a pharmacist, I know that a meta-analysis of several studies of antidepressants showed that patients taking drugs averaged a 40% drop in depression scores but the improvement is apparently at least 75% due to a placebo effect, indicating that medication is only 25% better than non-medication in the treatment of depression. I'm also worried about the side effects of antidepressants that commonly include:

- weight gain or loss
- reduced libido
- erectile dysfunction
- drowsiness
- dizziness
- urinary retention

- skin rashes
- stomach pain
- nausea
- diarrhea
- dry mouth
- sleep disturbances
- nightmares
- dry eyes
- anxiety
- worsened depression
- headache

"Plus rarer but potentially more serious adverse reactions like:

- suicidal thoughts
- interactions with certain drugs and foods causing dangerous hypertension
- seizures
- heart attack and stroke."

He went on. "I am particularly concerned about the possibility of stroke as a side effect of antidepressants, especially since my father died of one. There must be natural non-pharmaceutical measures I could supplement with in addition to the medications to lift my depression. I know you're not a psychiatrist, but you *are* a neurologist and I was hoping you could share your knowledge of the relationship between psychological imbalances and the increased risk of stroke, and whether there are any natural remedies that may alleviate the dangers altogether."

After telling my friend I was sorry to hear of his circumstances, I added, "You are correct to suspect that psychological disturbances contribute to the risk of stroke," and told him of the following studies that supported his concern:

- Professor Shah Ebrahim, stroke epidemiologist of the Department of Social Medicine at the University of Bristol and his colleagues reported in the results of their 14-year study of 2,124 men aged between 49-64 years old that subjects with a history of depression and anxiety were three times more likely to suffer a fatal stroke compared to participants who had no psychological distress.[149]

- Kimberly J. Salaycik and associates from Boston University School of Medicine reported in their eight-year study of 4,120 subjects less than 65 years old that the risk of developing stroke was 4.21 times greater in subjects with depression compared to non-depressed individuals.[150]

- European research by Dr. Martin Liebetrau and co-investigators followed 494 85-year-old subjects with and without dementia over three years and found an almost four-fold increase risk of stroke in depressed participants.[151]

- For 16 years, investigators from the Office of Analysis, Epidemiology and Health Promotion, National Center for Health Statistics, Centers for Disease Control and Prevention in the United States followed 6,095 stroke-free white and black men and women aged 25 to 74 years and found that depression increased the relative risk of stroke by 1.7 times in all groups.[152]

- A 10.3-year study of 901 Japanese men and women aged 40 to 78 by lead investigator Dr. Tetsuya Ohira found that subjects with depression—even if mild—

had two times the risk of suffering a stroke relative to their non-depressed cohorts.[153]

- Margaret May and co-investigators followed 2,124 men aged 49 to 64 for 14 years in the Caerphilly Study and reported that participants with depression were more than three times as likely to suffer a fatal stroke than comparable, non-depressed, middle-aged men.[154]

"I suspected as much," Mr. Notable told me. "The evidence of depression increasing the risk of stroke is most persuasive— but does anyone know why?"

"There are several plausible explanations for the association of depression and stroke," I replied, "including the reality that depressed individuals:

- have elevated inflammatory markers
- are notoriously non-compliant to treatments
- mostly lack exercise
- tend to smoke
- possess poor diabetes mellitus and hypertension control
- have heightened platelet aggregability
- practise unhealthy eating habits."

"Are there any natural strategies I can adapt that could help lift my depression?" Mr. Notable wondered next.

I answered that there were a few things he could try. Depression grows from discontent, which is a subjective perception that our wants and needs are not met. Despair may be resolved by returning to fundamentals. Be comforted that life's three basic essentials of food, shelter and clothing are easily found. The other two vital necessities of air and water are freely available.

Simplicity reduces our needs, diminishes our desires, minimizes our disappointments and maximizes our contentment, leading us to a life of serenity.

"Are you saying that we shouldn't aspire to improve our status in society?" questioned a puzzled Mr. Notable. For his entire life he had competed for material superiority over his peers.

"Absolutely not," I replied. "We should never cease to aspire to excellence but we must also be realistic so as not to feel despondent if we fail to achieve our objectives. We should be pleased with our endeavours even if we fail to attain our goals. Not everybody can be a president or an Olympian or a Nobel laureate, but that doesn't mean that we can't or shouldn't try for the honour. We must continue to strive with our best efforts to enhance our existence. It should be exhilarating enough that we meet this challenge," I encouraged.

"Don't you worry about what others think?" was Mr. Notable's next query.

"Well, we're only human," I answered him, but added that I had decided not to hold my happiness hostage to the approval of others. Each of us is an independent, distinct, separate, and unique person with our own genes, abilities, knowledge, beliefs, physique, appearance and experiences. I should not criticize others nor will I permit others' perceptions of my differences or individuality to influence my serenity, assuming that my eccentricities are not harmful, illegal, indecent or immoral.

Happiness is idiosyncratic. Happiness springs from self-satisfaction. For example, if it pleases me to smile and wave hello to everybody I meet or to wear a tuxedo while jogging, then I should not feel slighted if I overhear comments from passersby like "He's funny." On the contrary, I should be pleased that my existence is significant enough to be acknowledged by my fellow human beings. It would be more demeaning if my presence was so irrelevant as to be completely ignored.

"But what about the insult to your ego? Surely any self-respecting person would feel humiliated by such a disparaging ridicule," Mr. Notable went on.

"Only if I choose to perceive the remark negatively," I said.

Every interaction is, of itself, neutral. Whether an event is positive or negative depends on one's perception. Shakespeare states this truism succinctly in *Hamlet:* "... there is nothing either good or bad, but thinking makes it so."[155] For example, if it is raining when I wake up in the morning, I would feel frustrated if I had planned to jog that day. The downpour itself is neutral; it is my perception of the occurrence that is distressing. In other words, I have perceived the natural phenomenon negatively because it interfered with my plans for the day. On the other hand, I could easily change my mood 180° from displeasure to joy by thanking heaven for the rain that gives me a free day to finally read the book I haven't had time for. What changed my emotion from gloom to elation? Not the rain, which is still pouring. What is different is my attitude. I have adapted to reality.

Adaptability is the key to existence as witnessed by the survival of the fittest through natural selection: the most compliant organisms live and the unyielding creatures perish. A teacher once said that we should correct what is controllable and adapt to what is uncontrollable. And Lao Tzu teaches that "what is malleable is always superior to that which is immovable. This is the principle of controlling things by going along with them, of mastery through adaptation."

No human being has the ability to change a natural phenomenon, but all of us can control our responses to life's ever-changing circumstances. Affirmative thinking makes the difference. In short, always be positive. Every event has a negative and positive side.

"And life would a whole lot happier if we always chose the positive side of the equation," I told Mr. Notable.

"Sure, I can see how adapting to reality pertains to the present—but what about the past?" he asked. "We all know that the past is unchangeable, and lots of us have experiences we wish we could change. But what has happened can never be undone. How can the principle of positive adaptation be useful in the past?" my friend asked.

"Remember that the past is just a memory," I said, "and memories are illusionary remembrances subject to personal interpretation. We are what we think.

"Suppose you have lost a family member. You feel sad whenever you remember your loved one. But why do you feel despondent? Surely not because they are suffering—the liberated spirit is free of bodily concerns. It is more likely that the sense of loss itself is depressing you and the despondency is a result of negative thinking. You can easily change the memory of this past event from a recollection of sadness to an experience of joy by simply being thankful that your departed loved one is eternally serene. You have switched your thinking from negative to positive, and this ability to adapt can create powerful changes."

"But what about the future?" Mr. Notable wanted to know. "Don't you ever worry about what's to come?"

"'The past is eternal, the future is unending, the present is instantaneous,' my mother always said. What she meant can be understood by the following. Imagine the simple act of walking. As you step forward, your back leg is already in the past and your front is stepping about 1.5 feet and one second into the future. The present is the 1.5-foot distance (the *here*) and the one second between the time (the *now*) your back foot is on the ground and your front foot touches down. In that instant, the past is history and the future a reality, and unless you can travel at the speed of light, the present is forever gone. In that same moment, your space and time are different. Even *you* have changed. You are not the same person you were just a moment earlier. In that one split second, you have inhaled a certain amount of oxygen to fuel your energy needs, or exhaled a quantity of carbon dioxide, a by-product of your body's vital processes; your kidneys have excreted a fraction of a millimeter of urine, the waste product of metabolism; you have generated numerous fresh cells to replace exhausted ones and repaired a myriad of damaged tissues from nutrients provided by your last meal; your senses have perceived many experiences that are newly imprinted in your memory. You have physically, mentally, spatially and temporally adapted to a new reality. You might even argue that we can live only in the past since the present is simply the instantaneous passage to the future!

When you look into the night sky and admire bright, shining Polaris, you are actually seeing light that was emitted from the North Star 430 years ago. You are living a past event. When you smell the fragrance of a flower, you are experiencing a scent that was perceived by your nose and transmitted to your brain microseconds earlier, and interpreted by your nerve cells to be the perfume of a rose at the instant you are conscious of the pleasant sensation—but the experience has already been completed, even if just nanoseconds earlier.

The past is inescapable, the present irreversible and the future inevitable. It is the certain imminence of the future that necessitates a hoping-for-the-best-but-planning-for-the-worst kind of thinking, ensuring your personal contentment regardless of any eventuality. A wise man once observed that "Living is constant adaptation; sickness ensues if adaptation is restricted; life ceases when adaptation fails."

Anxiety and depression combined account for 16.2 of every 1,000 patient visits to doctors, second only to hypertension at 21. The economic cost of anxiety is estimated to be $46.6 billion US or 31.5% of total expenditures for mental illness in the United States in 1990. The total annual cost of depression in Europe was estimated in 2004 at €118 billion, which is equal to €253 per European.[156]

"So depression heightens the risk of stroke, but are other psychological stresses such as anxiety associated with an increased risk too?" inquired Mr. Notable.

"Yes," I told him. The following studies show that emotional distress elevates risk of stroke:

- An analysis of 20,627 stroke-free participants followed for 8.5 years by Dr. Paul Surtees at the University of Cambridge reported that the risk of stroke increases by 11% in psychologically distressed subjects.[157]

- Margaret May and colleagues in the United Kingdom answered affirmatively to the question "Does Psychological Distress Predict the Risk of Ischemic Stroke and Transient Ischemic Attack?" by showing a 1.45 times increase in the incidence of ischemic stroke in subjects with psychological distress in the Caerphilly Study of 2,201 men. The relative risk for fatal stroke was even higher, at 3.36 times that of non-psychologically distressed cohorts.[158]

- In a study of 600 acute stroke patients admitted to at Sahlgrenska University Hospital, neurologist Dr. Katarina Jood found that psychological stress is an independent risk factor for stroke.[159]

- Dr. Akizumi Tsutsumi of the University of Occupational and Environmental Health, Fukuoka, Japan and colleagues reported in their study of 6,553 Japanese workers followed for an average of 11 years the finding that labourers with high job stress (a combination of high job demand and low job control) suffered a more than two-fold increase in the risk of stroke compared to their counterparts with low job stress (a combination of low job demand and high job control).[160]

- Dr. William E. Haley and co-workers from the University of South Florida's School of Aging Studies found in their investigation of 676 caregivers that the psychological stress associated with caring for a disabled spouse can significantly increase the caregiver's risk of stroke, especially for African-American men, who experienced an estimated 26.9% increase in their 10-year risk for stroke.[161]

Fear is the emotional reaction to an immediate, actual threat whereas anxiety is a psychological response to an illusionary, imagined danger. *Fear that is realistic is protective since it alerts the threatened individual to "fight or flight" responses to actual menace, thereby ensuring survival.* For example, you are awakened from a nap by the smoke detector and realize that your house is on fire. This justifiable fright immediately mobilizes your sympathetic nervous system, providing you with the resources to fight or flee the actual catastrophe.

Conversely, *irrational fear, based on false beliefs, is destructive and even deadly.* Witness voodoo death. A witch doctor points a chicken bone at a transgressor. The cursed victim drops dead instantly. What happened? The fatality occurs not because of the disarticulated bird skeleton or the shaman's supposed powers. The true explanation is that the terrified victim was literally frightened to death. The fallacy of imminent doom releases a tsunami of a fight or flight hormone called *norepinephrine,* more commonly known as "stress hormone." **Norepinephrine** is a natural hormone crucial to the normal functioning of our body's stress defenses. However, a sudden surge of this vital sympathetic nervous system chemical is toxic—especially to the *myocardium,* the muscle of the heart, and essentially causes heart failure. In short, a lack of knowledge is dangerous to our survival.

Anxiety, especially if chronic, is harmful because the subjectively-generated, negative responses in reaction to misinterpreted, nebulous and intangible threats keep the body under constant tension, with a steady release of damaging stress hormones—including *cortisol, somatotropin* and *norepinephrine*—that permanently damage our physical and mental health. Anxiety results from unwarranted and exaggerated worry over misunderstood or imagined external threats," I told my friend.

"But what is the cause of anxiety?" Mr. Notable asked.

"There are several competing theories as to the cause of anxiety, including behavioral, developmental and biological," I answered. "But the simplest theory is the most logical. The cognitive theory proposes that anxiety, like fear, results from a lack of knowledge. To paraphrase Lao Tzu, 'He who knows, does not worry. He who worries, does not know.'

"But if anxiety results from a lack of wisdom or knowledge, as this theory suggests, then learning and studying should eliminate apprehension, isn't that true?" quizzed the pharmacist.

"It does appear that the theory validates the popular proverb 'Ignorance breeds fear. Knowledge drives those fears out,' leading us to the inescapable conclusion that learning is a principal natural remedy for anxiety," I replied.

"Besides knowledge, are there other non-pharmaceutical strategies to alleviate anxiety?" Mr. Notable wondered.

"It seems that education is the ultimate emancipator," I agreed, "but there are other promising natural antidepressants."

NATURAL ANTIDEPRESSANTS

- **Exercise**: There is substantial evidence that exercise is as effective as antidepressants in treating mild to moderate depression.[162] Possible explanations for the efficacy of exercise in depression are:

- the distraction from stressful situations
- a new confidence in self-control and self-discipline
- enhanced social interaction with fellow Partici-pACTIONers
- improved self-image
- the increased release of endorphins, which are *endogenous mood elevators* and painkillers (ie. the "runner's high")
- the euphoria of accomplishment.

- **Music**: Listening to or playing music maximizes relaxation and minimizes stress responses, resulting in an emotional state of tranquility. Furthermore, a study out of England found that listening to music can reduce depression by up to 25%.[163]

- **Meditation**: A large number of studies suggest that meditation may alleviate depression.[164]

- **Breathing**: Respiration is not only the most vital of all our bodily functions but is the single involuntary activity that we are able to consciously control. We can live for many days without food, a couple of days without water but only a few minutes without breathing. Beyond survival, Tai Chi and yoga masters have long taught many other health benefits of deep breathing, including the reduction of stress, normalization of blood pressure, promotion of relaxation and slowing of heart rate. Below is an outline of respiratory techniques taught by master practitioners of the ancient art of deep breathing:

- ° sit upright or lie down flat in a comfortable position
- ° relax all your muscles, starting from the toes and gradually rising to the head
- ° concentrate on your existence
- ° dismiss all interfering thoughts
- ° close your eyes
- ° focus on your breathing
- ° inhale slowly and deeply through the nose into your abdomen, with the tip of your tongue resting gently against the hard palate of your mouth
- ° exhale leisurely through an open mouth.
- ° continue this slow, deep abdominal breathing exercise for three to five minutes.

Then I added, "I know an ancient Chinese secret that incorporates exercise, music, breathing *and* meditation that can relieve anxiety and depression: **Tai Chi**, which is also known as 'moving meditation.'"

In Tai Chi exercise:

- the eyes look but do not see
- the ears hear but do not listen
- the mouth neither eats nor speaks
- the nose breaths but is not breathless
- the body exerts but is not exhausted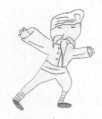
- the forms defend but do not offend
- the mind meditates, not cogitates
- the optional soothing music magnifies tranquility
- the flowing postures propel vital energies to rejuvenate each and every single one of the 50 trillion cells that compose the body.

"Tai Chi is the supreme healthercise," I enthused to Mr. Notable, who then asked if I knew of any other natural activities that could relieve emotional stress.

"Laughter!" I immediately replied. "As you know, it is the best medicine as validated by the French philosopher Voltaire's astute remark that 'the art of medicine consists of keeping the patient amused while nature heals the disease.'"

Scientists have proven that laughter:

- relieves physical tension and stress
- improves immunity
- releases endorphins that promote euphoria
- increases blood flow, preventing stroke and heart attack. Dr. Michael Miller of the University of Maryland School of Medicine found that blood flow in the major artery of the arm increased by 22% after normal volunteers watched a funny movie and decreased by 33% following the viewing of a distressing film, confirming that laughter improves circulation—probably by releasing endorphins that promote serenity
- dissolves anxiety, anger, depression, stress and tension
- provides health benefits equivalent to aerobic exercises. Laughing provides an excellent exercise for the whole body. Laughing intensely for 20 seconds is equal to 10 minutes on the rowing machine or 15 minutes on an exercise bike.[165]

"How can I laugh when there is so much conflict and hatred everywhere all the time?" Mr. Notable lamented.

"Easy. Just smile and laugh!" And remember to:

- Always look for the humorous side of any event.
  - Question: What happened to the man who lost the whole left side of his body?
    Answer: He's all right now. ~ANONYMOUS

- Focus only on the funny aspect of any situation.
  - "War does not determine who is right, war determines only who is left" ~BERTRAND RUSSELL

- Watch comedy TV programs and movies.
  - "*Three's Company* was originally called *Three Companies*, about a trio of pharmaceutical companies. It was 10 times funnier." ~JOHN RITTER

- Laugh with your friends.
  - You know you've got the greatest friends when the only time they make you cry is when you're laughing too hard. ~ANONYMOUS

- Surround yourself with funny people.
  - "Laughter is not at all a bad beginning for a friendship, and it is far the best ending for one."
    ~ OSCAR WILDE

- Learn to laugh at yourself.
  - "I am so clever that sometimes I don't understand a single word of what I am saying." ~OSCAR WILDE

  - "Laughing at our mistakes can lengthen our own life. Laughing at someone else's can shorten it."
    ~ CULLEN HIGHTOWER

  - "Never be afraid to laugh at yourself, after all, you could be missing out on the joke of the century."
    ~ DAME EDNA EVERAGE

- Keep on smiling. Like laughter, it's infectious.
  - "Laughter is the best medicine. Perhaps the biggest benefit of laughter is that it is free and has no known negative side effects." ~Anonymous

My reverie abruptly reverted to reality when I heard, "What are you smiling about?" from a totally unexpected but absolutely welcome source.

 Laughter and Serenity are the Best Medicine

- Simplify, simplify, simplify
- Learn limitlessly
- Persistently pursue positive adaptation
- Laugh your way to happiness
- Live in the moment
- Tai Chi healthercise daily.

13

stopping strokes saves lives

*"Physicians prescribe medicine of which they know little
to cure diseases of which they know less
to patients of whom they know nothing."*

~ VOLTAIRE

*"The doctor of the future will give no medicine,
but will educate his patients in the care of the human frame
in diet, and in the cause and prevention of disease."*

~ THOMAS A. EDISON

It was at 10:28 a.m. and I had just confirmed that the last drop of tPA had been infused into Mr. Patience's circulation. The blood pressure monitor read 168/88 and his pulse rate was 88 beats per minute. The auspicious 8s were adding up![a] I'd been thinking this was Mr. Patience's lucky day, which is why I was smiling.

"What are you smiling about?" Victor Patience repeated.

"I'm smiling because you lost the whole left side of your body, but everything's going to be all right now!" I reassured the rapidly convalescing stroke survivor.

a   In Chinese culture, 8 is a lucky number.

Laughter erupted as the intended pun sank in.

The crisis atmosphere around the critical care bed quickly evaporated as the joy of laughter dispersed the seriousness surrounding the emergency room.

"The Intensive Care Unit wants to know when Mr. Patience is being transferred there," said the ER ward clerk by the door. She wasn't sure what we were laughing about but her face broadened into a grin at the sound of our good spirits.

I smiled at her. "We are simply rejoicing that our stroke survivor here has been treated successfully with tPA. And please inform ICU that Mr. Patience is being moved there right now."

I was at home enjoying my customary fruit/vegetable salad dressed with plain yogurt, topped by ground flax seed and walnuts when the telephone rang. "Dr. Veloso, this is ICU," the caller announced as soon as I answered.

"What's happened? How's my patient?" were my immediate questions. In medicine I've found that, as is the case with so much else, no news is good news.

"Mr. Patience is doing well. He's conscious, talking and moving his arms and legs. His vital signs are stable and what's even more remarkable is that he is asking what's for supper. But his son, Patrick Patience, is here and wants to talk to you right away," the ICU nurse said.

"Thank you for the report; I'm glad to hear Mr. Patience is doing so well!" I heaved a great sigh of relief. "Please put Patrick Patience on the telephone."

"You don't understand. He wants to meet you personally, now, not just speak to you over the telephone," the nurse insisted.

"Kindly inform him that I'll be there in 15 minutes," I promised the harried nurse.

I rushed to Victor Patience's bedside as soon as I entered the ICU. I was just in time to overhear my patient say, "I have smoked my last cigarette!" to an athletic, casually dressed man in his late forties.

"Oh, hello, Dr. Veloso! I was just telling my son that I smoked my last cigarette this morning. Tomorrow will be the first day of the rest of my tobacco-free life!" Mr. Patience proudly proclaimed.

I was very pleased to hear it and told him so. "Are you all right? Can you move your arms and legs?" I questioned.

"I feel great. Oh! This is my son, Patrick, from Vancouver." Victor Patience pointed with his previously limp hand to the younger man standing beside his bed. I was greatly relieved to see positive proof that the paralysis had completely disappeared.

"Thank you so much for coming right away. I'm very sorry to interrupt your dinner, but I wanted to thank you personally for taking such good care of my dad before I go back to Vancouver on the last flight tonight," the smiling man apologized.

"Thank *you* for giving us permission to administer tPA to your father. Without your consent, we wouldn't have been able to treat his stroke successfully," I replied and continued, "You must be hungry. May I treat you and your mother to supper?"

"Thank you. I don't have enough time for supper but I'd love to have a cup of tea with you and my mother before going to the airport," said the doctor of pharmacy.

Mrs. Patience approached us from down the ICU hallway, chatting with another cheerful lady. "Dr. Veloso, this is Natalie Renaissance, the wife of the man who suffered a head injury in the car accident this morning," Mrs. Patience introduced her companion.

"Thank you for helping my husband," she said. "He's now asleep. The nurses say he's recovering nicely from the surgery. I'm so happy!" Mrs. Renaissance said, shaking my hand.

"Would you like to join us for tea?" I invited. Mrs. Patience and Mrs. Renaissance nodded their acceptance.

While sipping our green tea in the hospital cafeteria, Dr. Patience thanked me again for taking care of his father and then continued, "But I'm disappointed that it took a near-fatal stroke to cure my father of his 50-year-long, two-pack-a-day smoking habit. At the same time, I'm greatly relieved that he's finally quit. He's tried several stop smoking aids but found them all to be ineffective and loaded with side effects similar to—and some maybe even more serious than—tobacco itself. It appears that taking drugs to quit smoking only works if you're already determined to quit. Without the will, the weed will withstand."

"You must have a special interest in pharmacoeconomics," I mused. "What is your understanding of the cost benefits of other drugs commonly used to prevent stroke?"

"Well, I've analysed the cost-effectiveness of many recommended stroke prevention medications," he said, and added that:

- Taking cholesterol-lowering drugs is a lifetime commitment. Statistically, the chances of having a heart attack over the course of a lifetime are about 30% to 50% (higher for men than women). Studies sponsored by the pharmaceutical industry report **statins** reduce that risk by about 30%. But the trials of people without existing heart disease showed no reduction in either deaths or serious health events, despite the small drop in heart attacks. Nevertheless, statins have become the best-selling medicines in history, being used by more than 25 million patients worldwide at a cost of almost $28 billion US in 2006.[166]

- Are they cost-effective? A large clinical study over 40 months showed that 3% of patients taking a sugar pill or placebo had a heart attack, compared to 2% of patients taking a statin. This finding means that for every 100 people in the trial, which lasted 3.3 years, three people on placebo and two people on statin drugs had heart attacks—only one less heart attack per 100 people. In other words, to spare one person a heart attack, 100 people had to take a statin for more than three years. The other 99 got no measurable benefit. In terms of little-known but meaningful statistics, the *number needed to treat (NNT)* for one person to benefit is 100. Even worse, several later studies found the NNT for statins to be 250 or higher for low risk patients without pre-existing heart disease, even if they took the statin every day for five years or more at a cost of $1,000 per year.[167]

- This expense excludes the cost of management of known side effects of statins, including: muscle weakness, muscle pain, muscle cramps, liver damage, amnesia, confusion, disorientation, hostility, aggression, depression, fatigue, shortness of breath, diarrhea, heart failure and congenital malformation in about 38% of births from women who took cholesterol-lowering drugs during early pregnancy.[168]

- Furthermore, the nearly four-year Lyon Diet Heart Study found that a Mediterranean-style diet that emphasizes fruits, vegetables, cereals, bread, potatoes, beans, nuts, seeds, olive oil, dairy products, fish, poultry and moderate red wine reduces the risk of recurrent heart disease three times and the overall risk of death two times better than statin drugs.[169]

- Moreover, Dr. David Jenkins and fellow researchers at the University of Toronto and St. Michael's Hospital found in their month-long research of

46 men and women with raised cholesterol that a vegetarian diet composed of specific plant foods—including almonds, soy proteins, high-fibre foods such as oats, and margarine made with plant sterols found in leafy green vegetables and vegetable oils—can lower cholesterol as effectively as a statin drug.

The study found that a diet of known cholesterol-lowering vegetarian foods decreased low density lipoproteins (LDL or "bad cholesterol") by almost 29% compared to a 30.9% reduction from a standard cholesterol-reducing drug. The research also found that both the "portfolio" diets and the statin drug lowered *C-reactive protein (CRP)*, which is a marker of inflammation in the body linked to a higher risk of stroke and cardiovascular disease. The study recommends that people with high cholesterol should first try a "portfolio of cholesterol-lowering foods" before any statin drugs.[170]

- In a separate but related study, Dr. David Jenkins and his associates reported that both the cholesterol-lowering foods and a statin drug reduced C-reactive protein to a similar extent.[171]

- What's more, the National Health and Nutrition Examination Survey (NHANES) I Epidemiologic Follow-up Study[172] and other studies, including investigations by Dr. Ka He and associates from Harvard School of Public Health, found that higher consumption of fish and other omega-3 polyunsaturated fatty acids significantly reduces risk of stroke.[173]

- **C-reactive protein (CRP)** is a general marker for inflammation and infection. An elevated CRP has recently been associated with increased risk for heart attack and stroke. JUPITER, a new study of a widely prescribed statin, suggests that the cholesterol-lowering drug reduces the incidence of major cardiovascular events in normal cholesterolemic subjects with high blood CRP levels by 44%, compared to placebo. However, the more accurate statistics of absolute instead of relative risk reduction was far less impressive, being 1.36 bad outcomes per 100 person per years of follow-up in the placebo group, and 0.77 per 100 person per years in the statin group. This translates into a statin NNT of 120 over 1.9 years to prevent a cardiovascular disease event at a cost of $203,000 per event per year. It is important to remember that the JUPITER trial compares a proven cholesterol-lowering agent against a sugar pill.[b][174, 175]

- It is easier to understand why a five-year clinical trial involving 20,000 high stroke risk subjects comparing 81 mg of aspirin—the standard treatment for the prevention of strokes and heart attacks—against 81 mg of sugar was terminated prematurely at two years because interim analysis showed that aspirin is 100 times more effective than sugar in preventing major cardiovascular events.

Health care authorities could save their governments billions in drug costs alone by conducting a head-to-head trial of lifestyle modifications versus statins in the prevention of car-

---

b The JUPITER trial was prematurely terminated in the second of a planned five-year study when interim analysis showed that the statin was better than placebo.

diovascular events. Many experts believe that such a study may show that lifestyle modifications of a **Cretan/Mediterranean** type-**diet** and regular exercises may lower CPR and cardiovascular events similar to or better than statins but at much lower cost and without side effects.[176]

- It is worth remembering some of the feared serious side effects of statins, including *rhabdomyolysis, myopathy, peripheral neuropathy* and *diabetes mellitus*. The experts' conviction that a healthy lifestyle may reduce CRP and heart disease equal to statins is supported by various investigations:

  ◦ The study by E. S. Ford and colleagues from the Division of Environmental Hazards and Health Effects, National Center for Environmental Health, Centers for Disease Control and Prevention, Atlanta, Georgia found that C-reactive protein concentration was inversely and significantly associated with concentrations of *retinol, retinyl esters, Vitamin C, alpha-carotene, beta-carotene, cryptoxanthin, lutein/zeaxanthin, lycopene* and *selenium,* and concluded with the recommendation that the increased consumption of foods rich in antioxidants or supplementation with antioxidants can provide health benefits to people with elevated C-reactive protein concentrations and may be worthy of further study.[177]

  ◦ Simonetta Friso and associates from the Jean Mayer United States Department of Agriculture Human Nutrition Research Center on Aging at Tufts University, Boston, Massachusetts concluded that low *pyridoxal 5'-phosphate (PLP),* the active form of Vitamin B_6, is associated with higher CRP levels.[178]

○ S. Devaraj and I. Jialal from the Southwestern Medical Center, University of Texas reported that *α-Tocopherol*[c] therapy (Vitamin E therapy) decreases C-reactive protein in normal volunteers and reduces inflammation in Type 2 diabetic patients.[179]

○ In a related study, S. Devaraj and colleagues found that 1,200 IU of *α-Tocopherol* daily for two years significantly lowered high-sensitivity C-reactive protein concentrations by as much as 32% compared to placebo.[180]

○ J.E. Upritchard and co-investigators from the Department of Human Nutrition, University of Otago, Dunedin, New Zealand found that consumption of commercial tomato juice is almost as effective as supplementation with a high dose of Vitamin E in decreasing plasma levels of CRP, which is a risk factor for myocardial infarction in diabetic patients.[181]

○ G. Block and collaborators from the University of California, Berkeley reported that Vitamin C reduces median C-reactive protein (CRP) by 25.3% among participants with an elevated CRP of at least 1 mg/L, which is an effect similar to that seen with statins.[182]

---

c **Tocopherols (TCP)** are a series of organic chemical compounds of which many have Vitamin E activity. **Tocotrienols**, which are related compounds, also have Vitamin E activity. All of these various derivatives with vitamin activity may correctly be referred to as "Vitamin E." Tocopherols and tocotrienols are fat-soluble antioxidants but also seem to have many other functions in the body. http://en.wikipedia.org/wiki/Tocopherol. Accessed Nov. 10, 2010.

○ Dr. Dana King and co-investigators from the Medical University of South Carolina in Charleston reported that of 35 subjects who increased their dietary fibre intake from approximately 12 grams per day to between 27 to 28 grams daily reduced their pre-study C-reactive protein levels by 30 to 40% in just three weeks.[183]

○ The nearly four-year Lyon Diet Heart Study of 605 subjects who had heart attacks and randomized its subjects either to a Mediterranean-style diet (emphasizing fruits, vegetables, cereals, bread, potatoes, beans, nuts, seeds, olive oil, dairy products, fish, less red meat—which was replaced with poultry—as well as moderate red wine) or to a routine post-heart attack diet of reduced total and saturated fats, found that subjects following the Mediterranean-style diet had a 50% to 70% lower risk of recurrent heart disease, including less cardiac death and non-fatal heart attack, stroke, heart failure and pulmonary or peripheral embolism.[184]

○ A two-month study of 86 hyperlipidemic subjects at Kunming University in Southwestern China found that five grams of *Yunnan Tuocha* tea (a type of *pu-erh* tea) drunk three times daily lowers blood serum cholesterol by 64.29%, which is comparable to the 66.67% reduction produced by the standard cholesterol-reducing drug *Atromid-S Clofibrate Ethyl P-Cholorophenoxy-Isobutyrate* (PCIB).[185]

∘ Studies in the past 20 years have shown that those who daily consume about one to two ounces of soy protein for about four weeks can experience a decrease in their total and LDL cholesterol levels of as much as 10 - 20% when initial blood cholesterol levels are elevated. In some instances, those with normal blood cholesterol levels may also enjoy the benefit of lowered blood lipid levels by consuming soy. While LDL levels are decreased, HDL levels normally remain unchanged.[186]

∘ The use of soy also lowers triglyceride levels, especially in subjects with elevated blood triglyceride levels. The blood lipid responses tend to be more pronounced in younger adults than in older adults. These reductions are normally greater in subjects with high initial cholesterol levels. A recent meta-analysis of 38 controlled, clinical trials found that an average intake of 47 grams of soy protein per day produced, on average, a 13% decrease in LDL cholesterol levels and a 10% decrease in triglyceride levels.[187]

∘ As little as one to two ounces of isolated soy protein incorporated into muffins, breads, cookies and other commonly eaten bakery items can effectively lower the cholesterol levels of men who initially had cholesterol levels above 220 mg/dl.[d] Simply replacing milk with a soy beverage has been shown to cause blood cholesterol levels to decrease about 5 - 10% and LDL cholesterol levels to drop 10 - 20% within four weeks. It is obvious

---

d Milligrams per decilitre.

that very modest changes in diet appear to have a measurable effect on blood lipid levels.[188]

○ Though the precise way soy works is not known with certainty at this time, it is clear that soy isoflavones are potent inhibitors of cholesterol synthesis, and the plant sterols (for example, *beta-sitosterol*) and *saponins* in soy can block cholesterol absorption from the diet or increase cholesterol excretion from the body.[189]

○ Dr. Keri L. Monda of the University of North Carolina in a nine-year study of 9,000 sedentary middle-aged adults reported that each hour of moderate exercise, like taking a brisk walk, resulted in an almost 4-5.9 mg/dl reduction of LDL cholesterol in white women, and more than 10 - 14.68 mg for black women, with post-menopausal subjects achieving the higher LDL reduction.[190]

With regards to antihypertension drugs, a study by Dr. Jonathan T. Edelson and co-investigators evaluated the comparative efficacy and cost-effectiveness of various antihypertensive medications in people aged 35 through 64 years with diastolic blood pressure of 95 mm Hg or greater and no known coronary heart disease, and estimated that after 20 years of simulated therapy, the cost per year of life saved was projected to be the lowest using a beta-blocker—at $10,900, and the most expensive for an ACE inhibitor at $72,100. A calcium channel inhibitor was rated in the middle, at $31,600, suggesting that beta-blockers may be the preferred initial therapy for most patients with hypertension. But the cost of exercise to lower high blood pressure is practically nil and is completely without negative side effects, ranking physical activity as the most cost-effective treatment for most people with hypertension.[191]

The Dietary Approaches to Stop Hypertension (DASH) plan emphasizes eating fruits, vegetables and low-fat dairy products, high fibre, calcium, magnesium and potassium, and staying away from refined carbohydrates and saturated fats while minimizing daily salt intake to less than two grams. Individuals with mild hypertension on the DASH diet achieved a reduction in blood pressure similar to that obtained by drug treatment. The benefit is seen within two weeks of starting the plan.

Although those with hypertension lowered their blood pressure the most, those without hypertension also had big reductions in blood pressure. The DASH diet is easy to follow. Just double your fruit and vegetables, use low-fat dairy and cut your salt to two grams or less per day. Add spices and/or herbs to flavour your food instead. The DASH diet can also lower the risk of cancer, heart disease, diabetes and osteoporosis. If you are overweight, losing as little as 5 to 10% of your body weight can normalize your blood pressure and eliminate the need for prescription drugs.[192]

"I have also done some research regarding the cost-effectiveness of diabetic drugs," Patrick Patience went on.

- Jaakko Tuomi-lehto, professor at the National Public Health Institute in Finland showed in her study that people at high risk for developing Type 2 diabetes can reduce their chances of getting the disease by 58% through weight reduction, regular exercise and eating a healthy diet.[193]

- The Diabetes Prevention Program Research Group reported their findings that lifestyle intervention reduced the incidence of Type 2 diabetes by 58% versus the significantly less 31% provided by the anti-diabetic drug *metformin*, confirming that a healthy lifestyle is considerably more effective than diabetic medications. The same study also found that to prevent one case of diabetes during a period of three years, only 6.9 people needed to participate in the lifestyle-intervention program—less than half the 13.9 individuals that have to receive *metformin*.[194]

- Dr. William H. Herman and co-investigators reported their findings that lifestyle intervention was highly cost-effective, costing only $1,100 per quality adjusted life years, and that *metformin* intervention was much more expensive, costing approximately $31,300—confirming that lifestyle modification compared with *metformin* medication provided greater health benefits at a lower cost and should be the intervention of choice for the prevention of diabetes mellitus.[195]

Dr. Patience finished speaking, then asked, "What about you, Dr. Veloso, can you tell me about the cost-benefits of natural lifestyle changes in stroke prevention?"

Prudence Patience and Natalie Renaissance each took another sip of their green tea and looked at me with interest as well.

"Well, I know you have to go soon, but perhaps I will just mention that the 'Risk factors for ischaemic and intracerebral haemorrhagic stroke in 22 countries (the INTERSTROKE study): a case-control study' reported in the prestigious medical journal *The Lancet* their confirmation that the 10 risk factors of hypertension, smoking, obesity, unhealthy diet, physical inactivity, diabetes mellitus, alcohol abuse, stress and depression, heart disease and hyperlipedemia accounted for more than 90% of strokes—with the first five causes responsible for 80%, and the second five problems accounting for the other 10%."

My listeners shook their heads, astounded.

"But the most significant finding of the research," I went on, "is that all, and I repeat *all*, **the 10 risk factors for stroke can be neutralized by adopting a healthy lifestyle**. In other words, *90% of strokes are preventable by cost-free and side effect-free lifestyle changes*.[196] There is no medication I know of, regardless of price or side effects, that provides similar benefits."

"And what about the cost-savings of stroke prevention?" he wanted to know.

"Fifty thousand Canadians suffer a stroke every year, and 14,000 of them—just over 1 out of every 4—die from the brain attack. The latest estimate of the annual cost of caring for these stroke patients is at least $250 million a year, which is equivalent to $100,000 per victim.[197]

"The annual Canadian sales of just one of the many statin cholesterol-lowering drugs to prevent stroke is an estimated $1.1 *billion*. And that is the cost of just *one* medication used to prevent brain attacks, not including the amount of money spent on antihypertesive, anti-diabetic and antiplatelet drugs that are also widely prescribed to stop strokes. In striking contrast, *the cost of preventing stroke through natural, healthy lifestyle changes is zero*. Even the conservative estimate that a healthy lifestyle prevents only 50% of the annually reported 50,000 strokes (instead of the research-reported 90%), a healthy lifestyle still saves an invaluable 25,000 lives each year!—and the cost savings to our health care system is at least $100,000/patient, which, multiplied by 25,000 sufferers, equals a total of $2.5 *billion* in annual savings to our health care expenses," I replied.[198]

"You know, my husband has been depressed since recovering from a stroke he had two years ago," Mrs. Renaissance said. "He was prescribed antidepressants that likely contributed to the convulsion he experienced this morning. I am *so* relieved to hear you report that natural lifestyle changes can prevent 90% of strokes. Dr. Veloso, would you kindly summarize for us the natural, non-pharmaceutical lifestyle changes that so greatly reduce the risk of stroke?"

"Sure!" I responded. "Here is an overview of the natural lifestyle changes that can reduce the risk of suffering a stroke by up to 90%. Feel free to customize each of these methods to your individual circumstances. Your health will improve by adopting even one of these ideas, but the benefits will accumulate in direct proportion to the number of them you practise."

 Natural Lifestyle Principles to Prevent Stroke

- Normalize your blood pressure

- Consume a diet rich in fibre, fruits, vegetables, whole grain bread, lean white meats and low in sugar, salt, trans and saturated fats

- Commit to regular physical activity—30 minutes of moderate intensity dynamic exercise three to four days a week

- Moderate your alcohol consumption (two ounces of whiskey or two bottles of beer or two 8 oz. glasses of wine a day)

- Maintain an ideal body weight

- Reduce sodium intake to less than than 2,400 mg a day or less than one teaspoon of table salt per day
- Never smoke

- Smile and laugh your way to longevity
  "The gods too are fond of jokes." ~Aristotle

- Enjoy music regularly
"The power of music to integrate and cure ... is quite fundamental. It is the profoundest non-chemical medication."
~Neurologist Dr. Oliver Sacks, *Awakenings*

- Simplify your lifestyle to reach contentment and attain serenity

- Learn, learn, learn
"Education is the best provision for the journey to old age." ~Aristotle

- Eat small, oily fish three times weekly or take one gram of omega-3 fatty acids daily

- Practise good dental hygiene, including flossing, at least once a day

- Take 1,000 units of Vitamin D daily

- Live in the moment
"You must live in the present, launch yourself on every wave, find your eternity in each moment."
~Henry David Thoreau

- Adapt positively to any situation
"It is not the strongest of the species that survives, nor the most intelligent. It is the one that is the most adaptable to change." ~Charles Darwin

À votre santé!

notes

1   Philip Gorelick, M.D., M.P.H. "Primary Prevention of Stroke: Impact of Healthy Lifestyle." *Circulation*. American Heart Association. 2008; 118: 904-906.
2   C.L. Sudlow et al. "Thienopyridine derivatives versus aspirin for preventing stroke and other serious vascular events in high vascular risk patients." *Cochrane Database System Review*. 2009; Oct 7(4): CD001246.
3   Philip Gorelick, M.D., M.P.H.
4   C.L. Sudlow et al.
5   "Antiplatelet—combo therapy for prophylaxis is not good: new study." http://www.pubmedinfo.com/Clopidogrel.aspx. Accessed October 14, 2010.
6   Ara S. Khachaturian et al. "Antihypertensive Medication Use and Incident Alzheimer Disease: The Cache County Study." *Archives of Neurology*. May 2006; 63: 686-692.
7   http://heartdisease.about.com/library/weekly/aa081301a.htm and http://arthritis.about.com/od/vioxx/a/vioxxrecall.htm. Accessed September 29, 2010.
8   Walter Lewis, Ph.D., Memory Elvin-Lewis, Ph.D. *Medical Botany: Plants Affecting Human Health*. 2nd Edition. Wiley. 2003.
9   *The Vegetarian Times*. October 1988.
10 Michael Moore. *Medicinal Plants of the Pacific West*. Santa Fe, NM. Red Crane Press. 1993.
11 Audio-Digest Emergency Medicine. "Stroke Management." http://www.cme-ce-summaries.com/emergency-medicine/em2610.html. Accessed September 30, 2010.
12 Heart and Stroke Foundation of Canada. www.heartandstroke.com.
13 "Risk factors for ischaemic and intracerebral haemorrhagic stroke in 22 countries (the INTERSTROKE study): a case-control study." *The Lancet*. July 10, 2010; 376(9735): 112-123.
14 Dr. Mike Sharma. "The Canadian Stroke Network's Burden of Ischemic Stroke (BURST) study" presented at the Canadian Stroke Congress in Quebec City. June 8, 2010.
15 Yvonne Teuschl, Michael Brainin. "Stroke education: discrepancies among factors influencing prehospital delay and stroke knowledge." *International Journal of Stroke*. American Heart Association. June 2010; 5(3): 187–208.
16 Jeffrey L. Saver, M.D. "Time is Brain—Quantified." *Stroke*. American Heart Association. 2006; 37: 263.
17 t-PA Stroke Study Group. National Institutes of Health, National Institute of Neurological Disorders and Stroke. "Tissue plasminogen activator for acute ischemic stroke." *New England Journal of Medicine*. 1995; 333(24): 1581-1587,
18 "Mainstream Medicine Finally Catches on to the Risks of Taking a Daily Aspirin." http://

www.thehealthierlife.co.uk/natural-health-articles/heart-disease/aspirin-pycnogenol-poli-cosanol-heart-disease-prevention-03456.html. Accessed October 1, 2010.

19 "Foods that Naturally Thin the Blood." http://www.ctds.info/natthinners.html. Accessed October 1, 2010.

20 Peter M. Rothwell, M.D., Ph.D., F.R.C.P. Charles P. Warlow, M.D., F.R.C.P. "Timing of TIAs preceding stroke. Time window for prevention is very short." Neurology. 2005;64:817-820.

21 Henry J.M. Barnett, M.D. et al. "Benefit of Carotid Endarterectomy in Patients with Symptomatic Moderate or Severe Stenosis." The New England Journal of Medicine. 1998; 339: 1415-1425.

22 Kenneth E. S. Poole, B.M., M.R.C.P. et al. "Reduced Vitamin D in Acute Stroke." Stroke. American Heart Association. 2006; 37: 243.

23 Shang-Shyue Tsai, Ph.D. et al. "Evidence for an Association Between Air Pollution and Daily Stroke Admissions in Kaohsiung, Taiwan. Stroke. American Heart Association. 2003;34: 2612.

24 "Traffic-related air pollution tied to stroke death." http://www.reuters.com/article/idUS-TRE6352F520100406. Accessed October 8, 2010.

25 "Auto exhaust linked to thickening of arteries, possible increased risk of heart attack." http://berkeley.edu/news/media/releases/2010/02/08_university_basel.shtml. Accessed October 8, 2010.

26 "Prehypertension." http://www.knowyourdisease.com/treatment-of-prehypertension. html. Accessed October 8, 2010.

27 F. J. He, C.A. Nowson, G.A. MacGregor. "Fruit and vegetable consumption and stroke: meta-analysis of cohort studies." The Lancet. January 28, 2006; 367(9507): 320-6.

28 Natalia S. Rost et al. "Plasma Concentration of C-Reactive Protein and Risk of Ischemic Stroke and Transient Ischemic Attack: The Framingham Study." Stroke. American Heart Association. 2001; 32: 2575-2579.

29 Helen Hansagi, Ph.D. et al. "Alcohol Consumption and Stroke Mortality." Stroke. American Heart Association. 1995; 26: 1768-1773.

30 Luke 4:23.

31 William Ernest Henley (1849-1903). "Invictus." Book of Verses. 1888.

32 "Tobacco, Alcohol and Illicit Drugs Responsible for Seven Million Preventable Deaths Worldwide." National Drug Research Institute. db.ndri.curtin.edu.au/media. asp?mediarelid=40. Accessed October 20, 2010.

33 "Strange but True Facts and Statistics You Have No Business Knowing." NetScientia Web Concepts. www.netscientia.com/strange_facts.html. Accessed October 20, 2010.

34 "Health Effects of Secondhand Smoke." Smoking & Tobacco Use. Centers for Disease Control and Prevention. www.cdc.gov/tobacco/data_statistics/fact_sheets/secondhand_smoke/health_effects/index.htm. Accessed October 20, 2010.

35 Henry David Thoreau. "Where I Lived and What I Lived For." Walden; or Life in the Woods. Boston, Ticknor and Fields. 1854.

36 Richard Doll. Richard Peto. Jillian Boreham. Isabelle Sutherland. "Mortality in relation to smoking: 50 years' observations on male British doctors. British Medical Journal. June 26, 2004; 328(7455): 1519.

37 "What are the Benefits of Quitting Smoking?" www.quitsmokingsupport.com/benefits-printable.htm. Accessed October 20, 2010.

38 Rudolf Jaenisch, Adrian Bird. "Epigenetic regulation of gene expression: how the genome integrates intrinsic and environmental signals." Nature Genetics. 2003; 33: 245-254.

39 "African Americans and Stroke." National Stroke Organization. http://www.stroke.org/site/PageServer?pagename=AAMER. Accessed October 14, 2010.

40 Alan Joel. "Can Nutrition Change Our Genetics? No Doubt." http://ezinearticles. com/?Can-Nutrition-Change-Our-Genetics?-No-Doubt&id=3701787. Accessed October 14, 2010.

41 Biswanath Mitra, D. Guha, P.K. Gangopadhya. Neutrigenomics: A New Frontier. Bangur Institute of Neurology. Kolkata. 2003.

42 M. Kallela et al. "Familial Migraine with and without aura: clinical characteristics and co-occurrence." *European Journal of Neurology*. September 2001; 8(5): 441-449.

43 Paola Sebastiani et al. "Genetic Signatures of Exceptional Longevity in Humans." http://www.sciencemag.org/cgi/content/abstract/science.1190532. *Science*. July 1, 2010. Accessed October 14, 2010.

44 R. Hambrecht, C. Walther, S. Möbius-Winkler, et al. "Percutaneous coronary angioplasty compared with exercise training in patients with stable coronary artery disease: a randomized trial." *Circulation*. 2004; 109: 1371-1378.

45 Richard P. Donahue, Ph.D. et al. "Physical Activity and Coronary Heart Disease in Middle-Aged and Elderly Men: The Honolulu Heart Program." *American Journal of Public Health*. June 1988; 78(6): 683-685.

46 I-Min Lee, MBBS, ScD. et al. "Exercise and Risk of Stroke in Male Physicians." *Stroke*. American Heart Association. 1999; 30: 1-6. http://stroke.ahajournals.org/cgi/content/short/30/1/1. Accessed October 15, 2010.

47 F.B. Hu, et al. "Physical activity and risk of stroke in women." *Journal of the American Medical Association*. June 14, 2000; 283(22): 2961-2967. http://www.ncbi.nlm.nih.gov/pubmed/10865274. Accessed October 15, 2010.

48 Chong Do Lee, Ed.D. et al. "Physical Activity and Stroke Risk." *Stroke*. American Heart Association. 2003; 34: 2475-2481.

49 Ralph L. Sacco, M.D., M.S. et al. "Leisure-Time Physical Activity and Ischemic Stroke Risk: The Northern Manhattan Stroke Study." *Stroke*. American Heart Association. 1998; 29: 380-387.

50 D.K. Kiely et al. "Physical activity and stroke risk: the Framingham Study." *American Journal of Epidemiology*. 1994; 140: 608-620.

51 Richard F. Gillum et al. "Physical Activity and Stroke Incidence in Women and Men: The NHANES I Epidemiologic Follow-Up Study." *American Journal of Epidemiology*. The Johns Hopkins University School of Hygiene and Public Health. 1996; 143(9): 860-869.

52 E. Lindenstrom, G. Boysen. J. Nyboe. "Lifestyle factors and risk of cerebrovascular disease in women. the Copenhagen Heart Study." *Stroke*. American Heart Association. October 1993; 24: 468-1472.

53 J. Z. Willey, M.D., M.S. et al. "Physical activity and risk of ischemic stroke in the Northern Manhattan Study." *Neurology*. American Academy of Neurology. 2009; 73: 1774-1779.

54 Jacob R. Sattelmair M.Sc. et al. "Physical Activity and Risk of Stroke in Women." *Stroke*. American Heart Association. 2010; 41: 1243-1250.

55 "Adequate exercise may protect against brain diseases." iHealthBulletin News. http://ihealthbulletin.com/blog/special-reports/adequate-exercise-may-protect-against-brain-diseases/. Accessed October 15, 2010.

56 Fernando Gómez-Pinilla et al. "Voluntary Exercise Induces a BDNF-Mediated Mechanism That Promotes Neuroplasticity." *Journal of Neurophysiology*. November 1, 2002; 88: 2187-2195.

57 "Adequate exercise may protect against brain diseases." iHealthBulletin News. http://ihealthbulletin.com/blog/special-reports/adequate-exercise-may-protect-against-brain-diseases/. Accessed October 15, 2010.

58 "Adequate exercise may protect against brain diseases."

59 "Canadian Stroke Network." Government of Canada. http://www.nce-rce.gc.ca/NetworksCentres-CentresReseaux/NCE-RCE/CSN-RCCACV_eng.asp. Accessed October 16, 2010.

60 Julie Stokes and Joan Lindsay. "Major Causes of Death and Hospitalization in Canadian Seniors." http://www.phac-aspc.gc.ca/publicat/cdic-mcc/17-2/c_e.html. Accessed October 16, 2010.

61 "Statistics." Heart and Stroke Foundation. http://www.heartandstroke.com/site/c.iklQLcMWJtE/b.3483991/k.34A8/Statistics.htm. Accessed October 16, 2010.

62 "Moderate exercise prevents cancer: study." Union for International Cancer Control. http://www.uicc.org/general-news/moderate-exercise-prevents-cancer-study. Accessed October 16, 2010.
63 Robert F. Zoeller Jr, Ph.D. "Lifestyle in the Prevention and Management of Cancer: Physical Activity." American Journal of Lifestyle Medicine. September 2009; 3(5): 353-361.
64 Abby C. King et al. "Personal and Environmental Factors Associated with Physical Inactivity Among Different Racial-Ethnic Groups of U.S. Middle-Aged and Older-Aged Women." Health Psychology. 2000; 19(4): 354-364.
65 "Marathons lead to fewer road deaths." Globe and Mail. December 21, 2007. http://www.theglobeandmail.com/life/marathons-lead-to-fewer-road-deaths/article804385/. Accessed October 17, 2010.
66 "Health Care in Canada." Canadian Institue for Health Information. Statistics Canada. 2006. http://secure.cihi.ca/cihiweb/products/hcic2006_e.pdf. Accessed October 18, 2010.
67 Ibid.
68 "ParticipACTION, The Mouse That Roared: A Marketing and Health Communications Success Story." Canadian Journal of Public Health. May/June 2004; 95(2). http://www.usask.ca/archives/participaction/english/media/PDF/CJPH_95_Suppl_2_e.pdf. Accessed October 17, 2010.
69 Ruth E. Taylor-Pilae, R.N., C.N.S., M.N., Erika S. Froelicher, R.N., M.P.H., Ph.D., F.A.A.N. "The Effectiveness of Tai Chi Exercise in Improving Aerobic Capacity: A Meta-Analysis." Journal of Cardiovascular Nursing. January/February 2009; 19(1): 48-57.
70 "Tai Chi Chuan." http://frank.mtsu.edu/~jpurcell/Taichi/taichi.htm. Accessed October 17, 2010.
71 "Yang Style Tai Chi." www.chebucto.ns.ca/Philosophy/Taichi/. Accessed October 18, 2010.
72 "Postures of the Cheng Man-Ching Tai Chi Form." Patience T'ai Chi Association. www.patiencetaichi.com/public/109.cfm. Accessed October 18, 2010.
73 Henrik Stig Jørgensen et al. "Predicted impact of intravenous thrombolysis on prognosis of general population of stroke patients: simulation model." British Medical Journal. July 31, 1999; 319: 288.
74 Timothy J. Ingall, MB, BS, PhD, FAHA. "Time is Prime." Stroke. American Heart Association. 2009; 40: 2264-2265.
75 A. Bellisari. "Evolutionary origins of obesity." Obesity Reviews. 2008; 9(2): 165-180.
76 K. O'Dea. "Diabetes in Australian Aborigines: impact of the western diet and lifestyle." Journal of Internal Medicine. August 1992; 232(2): 103-117.
77 Will Dunham. "Gut chemical may inspire new way to fight obesity." Nov. 26, 2008. http://www.reuters.com/article/idUSTRE4AP7R620081126. Accessed October 19, 2010.
78 Frances Moore Lappé. "Like Driving a Cadillac." Diet for a Small Planet. New York: Ballantine Books. 1982. pp. 66-69, 71, 76, 78-79, 84, 462-465, 468.
79 Kenneth K. Carroll. Elizabieta M. Kurowska. "Soy Consumptions and Cholesterol Reduction: Review of Animal and Human Studies." The Journal of Nutrition. The American Society for Nutrition. 1995;125(3): 5945.
80 "The Thermic Effect of Food." http://www.caloriesperhour.com/tutorial_thermic.php. Accessed Oct. 19, 2010.
81 "Soy: Health Claims." http://www.keepkidshealthy.com/nutrition/soy_protein.html. Accessed October 20, 2010.
82 "Nutrition of soybean." http://vasatwiki.icrisat.org/index.php/Nutrition_of_soybean. Accessed October 20, 2010.
83 "Soybean." http://en.wikipedia.org/wiki/Soybean. Accessed October 20, 2010.
84 James W. Anderson, M.D. et al. "Meta-Analysis of the Effects of Soy Protein Intake on Serum Lipids." New England Journal of Medicine. 1995; 333: 276-282.
85 Frank M. Sacks, M.D. et al for the American Heart Association Nutrition Committee. "Soy Protein, Isoflavones and Cardiovascular Health." Circulation. American Heart Association. 2006;113: 1034-1044.

86   E.F. Fabiyi. "Soyabean Processing, Utilization and Health Benefits." *Pakistan Journal of Nutrition.* Asian Network for Scientific Information. 2006; 5(5): 453-457.

87   Bradley J. Willcox, M.D. et al. *The Okinawa Program: Learn the Secrets to Healthy Longevity.* New York., NY Three Rivers Press. 2001.

88   Kerrie B. Bouker. Leena Hilakivi-Clarke. "Genisten: Does it Prevent or Promote Breast Cancer?" Georgetown University. Washington, D.C. http://ehpnet1.niehs.nih.gov/members/2000/108p701-708bouker/bouker-full.html#pos. Accessed October 20, 2010.

89   "History of Tofu in China." http://www.asiarecipe.com/chitofu.html. Accessed October 20, 2010.

90   Julie Edgar. "Types of Teas and their Health Benefits." http://www.webmd.com/diet/features/tea-types-and-their-health-benefits. Accessed October 21, 2010.

91   Nikolaos Alexopoulos et al. "The acute effect of green tea consumption on endothelial function in healthy individuals." *European Journal of Cardiovascular Prevention and Rehabilitation.* June 2008; 15(3): 300-305.

92   "Health effects of tea." http://en.wikipedia.org/wiki/Health_effects_of_tea. Accessed October 21, 2010.

93   T. T. Yang. M. W. Koo. "Chinese green tea lowers cholesterol level through an increase in fecal lipid excretion." *Life Science.* 2000; 66(5): 411-423.

94   "Green tea." http://www.umm.edu/altmed/articles/green-tea-000255.htm. Accessed October 21, 2010.

95   "Tea." http://en.wikipedia.org/wiki/Tea. Accessed October 21, 2010.

96   "Green Tea Side Effects." www.cupofgreentea.com/green-tea-side-effects.htm. Accessed November 1, 2010.

97   Ibid.

98   Ibid.

99   "Cocoa Beans as a Superfood and a Major Source of Antioxidants." http://www.articlesbase.com/chocolate-articles/cocoa-beans-as-a-superfood-and-a-major-source-af-antioxidants-854471.html. Accessed October 21, 2010.

100 "Facts about Caffeine." http://www.xs4all.nl/~4david/caffeine.html. Accessed November 19, 2010.

101 Iris Shai, R.D., Ph.D. et al. "Dietary Intervention to Reverse Carotid Atheriosclerosis. *Circulation.* American Heart Association. 2010; 121: 1200-1208.

102 Leslie Beck. "Added sugars increase heart-disease risk." *The Globe and Mail.* Wednesday, April 21, 2010.

103 "Salt Comes Out in WASH." Canadian Stroke Network. http://www.canadianstrokenetwork.ca/wp-content/uploads/2010/04/newsletter14en.pdf. Accessed October 30, 2010.

104 "The DASH Diet Eating Plan." http://dashdiet.org/. Accessed October 30, 2010. *The Dash Diet Action Plan.* Northbrook, Illinois, USA: Amidon Press.

105 R. R. Croft. "How useful is weight reduction in the management of hypertension?" *Journal of the Royal College of General Practitioners.* October 1986.

106 "Framingham Heart Study." http://www.framinghamheartstudy.org/. Accessed October 31, 2010.

107 Jonathon Myers, Ph.D. "Exercise and Cardiovascular Health." *Circulation.* American Heart Association. 2003; 107: e2-e5.

108 "Simple handgrip exercise lowers blood pressure, McMaster University researcher." October 14, 2004. http://www.medicalnewstoday.com/articles/14963.php. Accessed October 31, 2010.

109 "University of Maryland School of Medicine study shows laughter helps blood vessels function better." http://www.umm.edu/news/releases/laughter2.htm. Accessed October 31, 2010.

110 "How much sodium do I need?" www.cbc.ca/health/story/2009/07/23/f-salt-reducing-health-risks.html. Accessed October 31, 2010.

111 Norm Campbell, M.D. "Dietary Sodium and the Health of Canadians." Miami, Florida, January 2009. http://www.paho.org/english/ad/dpc/nc/salt_mtg_can_campbell.pdf. Accessed October 31, 2010.

112 Pasquale Strazzullo et al. "Salt intake, stroke, and cardiovascular disease: meta-analysis of prospective studies." British Medical Journal. November 2009; 339: b4567.

113 "The Shakedown on Salt." Canadian Stroke Network. http://www.canadian-health.ca/2_2/stroke_e.pdf. Accessed October 41, 2010.

114 "Fats and sugars." Food Standards Agency. http://www.eatwell.gov.uk/asksam/healthydiet/fssq/. Accessed October 31, 2010.

115 Glen Doucet, B.A. Margaret Beatty, R.N. M.H.Sc., C.H.E. "The Cost of Diabetes in Canada: The Economic Tsunami." Canadian Journal of Diabetes. March 2010; 34(1): 27-29.

116 "Type 2 Diabetes." http://en.wikipedia.org/wiki/Diabetes_mellitus_type_2. Accessed November 3, 2010.

117 Jaana Lindström, Ph.D. et al. "The Finnish Diabetes Prevention Study." Diabetes Care. American Diabetes Association. http://care.diabetesjournals.org/content/26/12/3230.abstract. Accessed November 3, 2010.

118 Anne-Helen Harding, Ph.D. et al. "Plasma Vitamin C Level, Fruit and Vegetable Consumption, and the Risk of New-Onset Type 2 Diabetes Mellitus." Archives of Internal Medicine. 2008; 168(14): 1493-1499.

119 L.A. Bazzano, T.Y. Li, K.J. Joshipura, F.B. Hu. "Intake of fruit, vegetables and fruit juices, and risk of diabetes in women." Diabetes Care. American Diabetes Association. 2008 Jul; 31(7): 1311-1317.

120 Rui Jiang et al. "Nut and Peanut Butter Consumption and Risk of Type 2 Diabetes in Women." Journal of the American Medical Association. 2002; 288(20): 2554-2560.

121 Julie R. Palmer, Sc.D. et al. "Sugar-Sweetened Beverages and Incidence of Type 2 Diabetes Mellitus in African American Women." Archives of Internal Medicine. 2008; 168(14): 1487-1492.

122 Leslie Beck. "Beans: good for your heart—and blood sugar." The Globe & Mail. http://www.theglobeandmail.com/life/health/good-for-your-heart-and-blood-sugar/article1241208/. Accessed November 3, 2010.

123 The Glycemic Index. http://www.glycemicindex.com/. Accessed November 3, 2010.

124 Diabetes Prevention Program Research Group. "Reduction in the Incidence of Type 2 Diabetes with Lifestyle Intervention or Metformin." New England Journal of Medicine. 2002; 346:393-403.

125 X.R. Pan et al. "Effects of diet and exercise in preventing NIDDM in people with impaired glucose tolerance. The Da Qing IGT and Diabetes Study." Diabetes Care. American Diabetes Association. 1997; 20(4): 537-544.

126 Allen J. Taylor, M.D. et al. "Extended-Release Niacin or Ezetimibe and Carotid Intima–Media Thickness." The New England Journal of Medicine. November 26, 2009; 361(22): 2113-2122.

127 Anthony Colpo. "LDL Cholesterol: 'Bad' Cholesterol, or Bad Science?" Journal of American Physicians and Surgeons. 2005; 10(3): 83-87.

128 R.H. Bradford et al. "Expanded Clinical Evaluation of Lovastatin (EXCEL) study results. Efficacy in modifying plasma lipoproteins and adverse event profile in 8245 patients with moderate hypercholesterolemia." Archives of Internal Medicine. 1991;151:43-49.

129 Paul M Ridker, M.D. "Rosuvastatin to Prevent Vascular Events in Men and Women with Elevated C-Reactive Protein." New England Journal of Medicine. 2008; 359: 2195-2207.

130 J. A. Welsh et al. "Caloric Sweetener Consumption and Dyslipidemia Among US Adults." The Journal of the American Medical Association, 2010; 303(15): 1490.

131 "William Osler." http://en.wikipedia.org/wiki/William_Osler. Accessed November 5, 2010.

132 "Heliobacter pylori." http://en.wikipedia.org/wiki/Helicobacter_pylori. Accessed November 5, 2010.

133 Yasunori Sawayama et al. "Association between chronic Helicobacter pylori infection and acute ischemic stroke: Fukuoka Harasanshin Atherosclerosis Trial (FHAT)." *Atherosclerosis.* 2005; 178: 303–309.

134 "Oral Health, U.S. 2002 Annual Report." The Dental, Oral, and Craniofacial Data Resource Center. http://drc.hhs.gov/report/3_1.htm. Accessed November 5, 2010.

135 K.J. Mattila et al. "Association between dental health and acute myocardial infarction." *British Medical Journal.* 1989; 298: 779.

136 Lorelei A. Mucci et al. "Do Genetic Factors Explain the Association Between Poor Oral Health and Cardiovascular Disease? A Prospective Study Among Swedish Twins." *American Journal of Epidemiology.* 2009; 170(5): 615-621.

137 Yukihito Higashi et al. "Periodontal Infection Is Associated With Endothelial Dysfunction in Healthy Subjects and Hypertensive Patients." *Hypertension.* 2008; 51:446-453.

138 Pirkko J. Pussinen et al. "Endotoxemia, Immune Response to Periodontal Pathogens, and Systemic Inflammation Associate With Incident Cardiovascular Disease Events." *Arteriosclerosis, Thrombosis, and Vascular Biology.* 2007; 27: 1433-1439.

139 Axel Spahr, D.D.S. et al. "Periodontal Infections and Coronary Heart Disease: Role of Periodontal Bacteria and Importance of Total Pathogen Burden in the Coronary Event and Periodontal Disease (CORODONT) Study." *Archives of Internal Medicine.* 2006; 166(5): 554-559.

140 C.E. Dörfer. "The association of gingivitis and periodontitis with ischemic stroke." *Journal of Evidence-Based Dental Practices.* 2005; 5(2): 92-93.

141 Steven P. Engebretson, D.M.D., M.S. "Radiographic Measures of Chronic Periodontitis and Carotid Artery Plaque." *Stroke.* American Heart Association. 2005; 36: 561-566.

142 Kaumudi J. Joshipura, Sc.D. et al. "Periodontal Disease, Tooth Loss, and Incidence of Ischemic Stroke." *Stroke.* American Heart Association. 2003; 34: 47-52.

143 "Atherosclerosis Risk in Communities (ARIC) Study." *American Journal of Epidemiology.* 1989; 129(4): 687-702.

144 Armin J. Grau, M.D. "Periodontal Disease as a Risk Factor for Ischemic Stroke." *Stroke.* American Heart Association. 2004; 35: 496-501.

145 Tiejian Wu et al. "Periodontal disease and risk of cerebrovascular disease: the first national health and nutrition examination survey and its follow-up study." *Archives of Internal Medicine.* 2000; 160(18): 2749-2755.

146 S.J. Sim et al. "Periodontitis and the risk for non-fatal stroke in Korean adults." *Journal of Periodontology.* 2008; 79(9): 1652-1658.

147 Henry David Thoreau.

148 Ibid.

149 Shah Ebrahim et al. "Does Psychological Distress Predict the Risk of Ischemic Stroke and Transient Ischemic Attack? The Caerphilly Study." *Stroke.* American Heart Association. 2002; 33: 7-12.

150 Kimberly J. Salaycik, M.A et al. "Depressive Symptoms and Risk of Stroke: The Framingham Study." *Stroke.* American Heart Association. 2007; 38: 16-21.

151 Martin Liebetrau, M.D. et al. "Depression as a Risk Factor for the Incidence of First-Ever Stroke in 85-Year-Olds." *Stroke.* American Heart Association. 2008; 39: 1960-1965.

152 Bruce S. Jonas, Sc.M., Ph.D. and Michael E. Mussolino, M.A. "Symptoms of Depression as a Prospective Risk Factor for Stroke." *Psychosomatic Medicine.* American Psychosomatic Society. 2000; 62:463-471.

153 Tetsuya Ohira, M.D. et al. "Prospective Study of Depressive Symptoms and Risk of Stroke Among Japanese." *Stroke.* American Heart Association. 2001; 32: 903-908.

154 Margaret May, M.Sc. et al. "Does Psychological Distress Predict the Risk of Ischemic Stroke and Transient Ischemic Attack? The Caerphilly Study." *Stroke.* American Heart Association. 2002; 33: 7-12.

155 William Shakespeare. *Hamlet.* Act 2, Scene 2.

156 P. Sobocki et. al. "Cost of Depression in Europe." *Journal of Mental Health Policy Economics.* 2006; 9(2): 87-98.

157 P.G. Surtees, Ph.D. "Psychological distress, major depressive disorder, and risk of stroke." *Neurology*. American Academy of Neurology. 2008; 70(10); 788-794.

158 Margaret May, M.Sc. et al.

159 Katarina Jood et al. "Self-perceived psychological stress and ischemic stroke: a case-control study." *BMC Medicine*. BioMed Central. 2009; 7:53.

160 Akizumi Tsutsumi, M.D. et al. "Prospective Study on Occupational Stress and Risk of Stroke." *Archives of Internal Medicine*. 2009; 169(1):56-61.

161 William E. Haley. Beth Han. "Family Caregiving for Patients With Stroke: Review and Analysis." *Stroke*. American Heart Association. 1999; 30: 1478-1485.

162 Marleen H. M. De Moor, M.Sc. et al. "Testing Causality in the Association Between Regular Exercise and Symptoms of Anxiety and Depression." *Archives of General Psychiatry*. 2008; 65(8): 897-905.

163 Sandra L. Siedlecki, M.D. "Listening to music can reduce chronic pain and depression by up to a quarter." *Journal of Advanced Nursing*. May 2006.

164 "Reduced depression with Transcendental Meditation?" http://integral-options.blogspot.com/2010/04/reduced-depression-with-transcendental.html. Accessed November 10, 2010.

165 "Laugh and the World Laughs With You..." *New Options for Wellness News*. SLAC Medical Department. Stanford Linear Accelerator Center. April/May 2005.

166 Tom Jacobs. "Cholesterol Contrarians Question Cult of Statins." *Miller-McCune*. 2009. http://www.miller-mccune.com/health/cholesterol-contrarians-question-cult-of-statins-3808/. Accessed November 10, 2010.

167 John Carey. "Do Cholesterol Drugs Do Any Good?" *BusinessWeek*. January 28, 2008.

168 R.J. Edison. M. Muenke. "Central nervous system and limb anomalies in case reports of first-trimester statin exposure." *New England Journal of Medicine*. 2004; 350(15):1579-1582.

169 Penny Kris-Etheron, Ph.D, R.D. et al. "Lyon Diet Heart Study: Benefits of a Mediterranean-Style, National Cholesterol Education Program/American Heart Association Step I Dietary Pattern on Cardiovascular Disease." *Circulation*. American Heart Association. 2001; 103: 1823.

170 David J.A. Jenkins et al. "Effects of a Dietary Portfolio of Cholesterol-Lowering Foods vs Lovastatin on Serum Lipids and C-Reactive Protein." *Journal of the American Medical Association*. 2003; 290(4): 502-510.

171 D.J. Jenkins et al. "Direct comparison of dietary portfolio vs statin on C-reactive protein." *European Journal of Clinical Nutrition*. 2005; 59(7): 851-860.

172 National Health and Nutrition Examination Survey: NHANES I Epidemiologic Followup Study (NHEFS). Centers for Disease Control and Prevention. http://www.cdc.gov/nchs/nhanes/nhefs/nhefs.htm. Accessed November 10, 2010.

173 Ka He, M.D., Sc.D. et al. "Fish Consumption and Incidence of Stroke: A Meta-Analysis of Cohort Studies." *Stroke*. American Heart Association. 2004; 35: 1538-1542.

174 Robert L. Ohsfeldt et al. "Cost effectiveness of rosuvastatin in patients at risk of cardiovascular disease based on findings from the JUPITER trial." *Journal of Medical Economics*. 2010; 13(3); 428-437.

175 Dr. Julian Whitake. "Cardiovascular Health and CRP: Statins Are Not the Answer." *Dr. Julian Whitaker's Health & Healing*, 2009; 19(1).

176 D.J. Becker et al. "Simvastatin vs therapeutic lifestyle changes and supplements: randomized primary prevention trial." *Mayo Clinic Proceedings*. 2008; 83(7): 758-764.

177 E.S. Ford. et al. "C-reactive protein concentration and concentrations of blood vitamins, carotenoids, and selenium among United States adults." *European Journal of Clinical Nutrition*. 2003; 57(9): 1157-1163.

178 Simonetta Friso, M.D. et al. "Low Circulating Vitamin B6 Is Associated With Elevation of the Inflammation Marker C-Reactive Protein Independently of Plasma Homocysteine Levels." *Circulation*. American Heart Association. 2001; 103: 2788-2791.

179 Sridevi Devaraj, Ph.D. et al. "α-Tocopherol Supplementation Decreases Plasminogen Activator Inhibitor-1 and P-Selectin Levels in Type 2 Diabetic Patients." *Diabetes Care*. American Diabetes Association. 2002; 25(3): 524-529.

180 Sridevi Devaraj, Ph. D. et al. "Effect of high-dose α-tocopherol supplementation on bio-markers of oxidative stress and inflammation and carotid atherosclerosis in patients with coronary artery disease." *American Journal of Clinical Nutrition.* 2007; 86(5):1392-1398.

181 J.E. Upritchard et al. "Effect of supplementation with tomato juice, vitamin E, and vitamin C on LDL oxidation and products of inflammatory activity in type 2 diabetes." *Diabetes Care.* American Diabetes Association. 2000; 23(6): 733-738.

182 G. Block et al. "Vitamin C treatment reduces elevated C-reactive protein." *Free Radical Biology & Medicine.* 2009; 46(1): 70-77.

183 Dana E. King, M.D., M.S. "Effect of a High-Fiber Diet vs a Fiber-Supplemented Diet on C-Reactive Protein Level." *Archives of Internal Medicine.* 2007; 167(5): 502-506.

184 Penny Kris-Etheron, Ph.D, R.D. et al.

185 "Research Studies on Yunnan Tuocha Tea." http://www.tuochatea.com/research.htm. Accessed November 10, 2010.

186 J. Anderson et al. "Meta-analysis of the effects of soy protein intake on serum lipiods." *New England Journal of Medicine.* 1995; 333: 276-82.

187 J. Anderson et al.

188 S. M. Potter et al. "Depression of plasma cholesterol in men by consumption of baked products containing soy protein." *American Journal of Clinical Nutrition.* 1993; 58: 501-506.

189 S. M. Potter et al. "Overview of proposed mechanisms for the hypocholesterolemic effect of soy." *Journal of Nutrition.* 1995;125:606S-11S.

190 Keri L. Monda, Ph.D. et al. "Longitudinal impact of physical activity on lipid profiles in middle-aged adults: the Atherosclerosis Risk in Communities (ARIC) Study." *Journal of Lipid Research.* 2009; 50(8): 1685-1691.

191 Jonathan T. Edelson, M.D. et al. "Long-term Cost-effectiveness of Various Initial Mono-therapies for Mild to Moderate Hypertension." *Journal of the American Medical Association.* 1990; 263(3): 407-413.

192 Thomas J. Moore et al. "DASH (Dietary Approaches to Stop Hypertension) Diet Is Effec-tive Treatment for Stage 1 Isolated Systolic Hypertension." *Hypertension.* American Heart Association. 2001; 38: 155-158.

193 Jaako Tuomi-lehto. "Prevention of Type 2 Diabetes Mellitus by Changes in Lifestyle." *New England Journal of Medicine.* 2001; 344:1343-1350.

194 Diabetes Prevention Program Research Group. "Reduction in the Incidence of Type 2 Diabetes with Lifestyle Intervention or Metformin." *New England Journal of Medicine.* 2002; 346: 393-403.

195 William H. Herman, M.D., M.P.H. et al. "The Cost-Effectiveness of Lifestyle Modification or Metformin in Preventing Type 2 Diabetes in Adults with Impaired Glucose Tolerance." *Annals of Internal Medicine.* 2005; 142(5): 323-332.

196 Martin J. O'Donnell, Ph.D. et al. "Risk factors for ischaemic and intracerebral haemor-rhagic stroke in 22 countries (the INTERSTROKE study): a case-control study." *The Lancet.* 2010; 376(9735): 112-123.

197 "Strokes cost Canada $2.5B a year: study." CBC News. Monday, June 7, 2010. http://www.cbc.ca/health/story/2010/06/07/stroke-cost.html?ref=rss. Accessed November 12, 2010.

198 Scott Anderson. Ransdell Pierson. "UPDATE 3-Lipitor generics reach Canada, Pfiz-er vows fight." Wednesday, May 19, 2010. Reuters. http://www.reuters.com/article/idUSN1924176320100519. Accessed November 10, 2010.

glossary

Adrenaline. A natural substance in the body that increases heart rate, narrows blood vessels and opens up air passages. Another name for epinephrine.

Aggrenox. A drug that inhibits blood clotting and widens blood vessels.

Alpha-adrenergic receptors. *(α-adrenergic receptors).* A receptor in cell membranes sensitive to the sympathetic adrenaline and noradrenadine hormones. Stimulation of alpha-adrenergic receptors increases blood pressure and inhibition of the receptors lowers blood pressure.

Alzheimer's disease. The most common cause of dementia in older adults.

Amaurosis fugax (Transient monocular blindness, TMB). A temporary loss of vision due to a partial or complete blockage of one of the two carotid arteries in the neck supplying the brain.

Amino acids. Organic molecules that are the building blocks of proteins.

Amyloid plaque. Aggregates of amyloid-beta in the brain in those who suffer from Alzheimer's disease.

Anaerobic. Without oxygen.

Ancrod. A potent natural anticoagulant derived from snake venom. Ancrod works by reducing blood levels of *fibrinogen*, a critical agent in blood clotting.

Anemia. A deficiency of red blood cells.

Angina. A heart condition marked by paroxysms of chest pain due to reduced oxygen to the heart.

Angioplasty. An operation in which a blocked artery is opened with a balloon.

Angiotensin converting enzyme (ACE) inhibitors. Drugs used to treat high blood pressure and congestive heart failure.

Angiotensin recepter blockers. Drugs used to treat high blood pressure, heart failure and to prevent kidney failure in people with diabetes or high blood pressure. They may reduce the risk of stroke. ARBs are similar to ACE inhibitors, and are often used when ACE inhibitors are not tolerated by the patient.

Anticoagulant. Compounds that inhibit blood clotting.

Anticonvulsant. Medication that prevents seizures.

Antigen. A substance capable of eliciting an immune response.

Antihypertensive. A substance that reduces high blood pressure.

Antioxidant. Molecules that prevent damage caused by reactive oxidizing agents.

Antiplatelet agent. A medication that helps prevent blood clotting.

Apoptosis. Gene-directed cell death or programmed cell death.

Arrhythmia. An irregular heart rhythm.

Arterial puncture. The wound created when a needle punctures an artery to draw blood.

Arteriovenous malformation. An abnormal connection between veins and arteries.

Arteriosclerosis. A hardening of the arteries due to the accumulation of plaque.

Atherosclerosis. An inflammation leading to the accumulation of cholesterol-laden plaque in artery walls.

Atrial fibrillation. A cardiac arrhythmia characterized by uncoordinated beating of the atria.

Autoimmune disease. A sickness in which the body's immune system reacts against its own tissues.

Bacteria. Single-celled organisms.

Brain-derived neurotrophic factor (BDNF). A nerve cell growth factor that supports the repair, growth, function and survival of neurons.

Bioavailability. The fraction of an administered compound free to act.

Blood pressure. Normal blood pressure is usually said to be 120/80 (systolic/diastolic) or less, measured in millimeters of mercury (abbreviated as mm Hg). The higher (systolic) number represents the pressure while the heart is beating. The lower (diastolic) number represents the pressure when the heart is resting between beats. The systolic pressure is always stated first and the diastolic pressure second.

Body Mass Index (BMI). A measure of weight in relation to height; to calculate your BMI, multiply your weight in pounds and divide that by the square of your height in inches; overweight is a BMI greater than 25; obese is a BMI greater than 30.

Brain stem. The part of the brain where the vital centres of respiration, heart rhythm, blood pressure, wakefulness, arousal, eye movement and attention are located.

Bruit. A swishing sound heard with a stethoscope over a partially blocked artery.

C-reactive protein (CRP). A protein that is a marker of inflammation.

CAT (CT) scan. (Computerized Axial Tomography). Pictures of structures in the body created by a computer with data from multiple X-rays.

Calorie. There are two forms of calories, both of which are units of heat energy. The "small" or "gram" calorie—the amount of energy needed to heat one gram of water by one degree Celsius—is used often in science, but is too small to conveniently describe the energy content of food, so the "kilocalorie" is used instead and is, confusingly, called simply a calorie in dietary terminology. The "food" calorie equals 1000 "gram" calories. The food or "kilogram" calorie represents the amount of energy needed to raise the temperature of a kilogram of water by one degree. Any mention of "calorie" in this book refers to the larger "food" calorie.

Carbohydrate. A macronutrient that provides a significant source of calories in the diet.

Cardiovascular. Referring to the heart and blood vessels.

Cardiovascular disease. Diseases of the heart and blood vessels.

Carotid arteries. The principal blood vessels supplying oxygenated blood to the head and neck. Each has two main branches with the *external carotid artery* providing the head and neck, and the *internal carotid artery* delivering to the brain.

Carotid endarterectomy. A surgical procedure in which the *stenosis*, or abnormal narrowing, of a carotid artery is corrected.

Carotid vessel wall volume. A measurement of atherosclerosis.

Case-control study. A study in which subjects who have been diagnosed with a disease are compared to volunteers without the disease (controls).

Case reports. Individual observations based on small numbers of subjects.

Catalyst. A substance that increases the speed of a chemical reaction.

Catecholamines. Hormones of the sympathetic nervous system such as *epinephrine* and *norepinephrine*.

Central nervous system (CNS). The brain, spinal cord.

Cerebellum. The part of the brain located behind the cerebrum repsonsible for balance and coordination.

Cerebral hemorrhage. A subtype of *intracranial hemorrhage*. Bleeding within the brain tissue.

Cerebrospinal fluid. The fluid that bathes the brain and spinal cord.

Cerebrovascular disease. A disease involving the blood vessels that supply the brain, such as a stroke.

Cerebrum. The largest part of the brain responsible for higher mental functions like intelligence, emotion, memory and speech.

Chagra. Dried brewed tea leaves.

Cholesterol. A compound needed for cell membranes and a precursor of steroid hormones.

Cholinergic. Releasing or activated by *acetylcholine*, a parasympathetic neurotransmitter.

Chromosome. A structure in the nucleus of cells that contains genes.

Chronic disease. An illness lasting for at least three months.

Chylomicrons. Triglyceride-rich *lipoproteins* that deliver dietary *triglycerides* from the intestine to the tissues immediately after a meal.

Clinical trial. A research designed to evaluate the usefulness and/or safety of a treatment or intervention in human participants.

Clopidogrel. Medication intended to help prevent blood clotting.

Coagulation. The blood clotting process.

Cognitive. An adjective referring to thinking, learning, perception, awareness and judgment.

Cohort study. A study following a large group of people over a long period of time.

Congestive heart failure. The inability of the heart to circulate blood adequately.

Coronary artery. A vessel that supplies oxygenated blood to the heart muscle.

Coronary artery bypass graft (CABG). A surgery to create new routes around a blockage in the coronary arteries to restore adequate blood flow to the heart muscle.

Coronary heart disease (CHD). *Atherosclerosis* of the coronary arteries. The number one killer in Canada.

Coronary insufficiency. Inadequate blood flow through one or more of the heart's arteries.

Corticosteroid. Any of the steroid hormones made by the cortex of the adrenal gland.

Cortisol. A stress hormone manufactured by the adrenal and pituitary glands.

Cytokine. A cellular protein that affects the behaviour of other cells.

Dementia. Significant impairment of intellectual abilities, such as attention, orientation, memory, judgment or language.

Dental caries. Cavities in the outer two layers of a tooth.

Diabetes mellitus. A metabolic disease characterized by abnormally high blood sugar levels resulting from the inability of the body to produce or respond to insulin.

Diastolic blood pressure. The lower number in a blood pressure reading (e.g. 120/80) representing the lowest arterial blood pressure during the heartbeat cycle.

Diuretic. Commonly known as a "water pill," an agent that increases the formation of urine by the kidneys.

DNA. The abbreviation for *deoxyribonucleic acid,* a double-stranded nucleic acid composed of many nucleotides. DNA encodes the genetic information required to synthesize proteins.

Dominant trait. A trait that is expressed when only one copy of the gene responsible for the trait is present.

Double blind study. A study in which neither the investigators administering the treatment nor the participants know which participants are receiving the experimental treatment and which are receiving the placebo.

Dyslipidemia. An abnormal amount of lipids (fat and/or cholesterol) in the bloodstream.

Edema. The accumulation of excessive fluid in tissues beneath the skin.

Eicosanoids. Chemical messengers derived from long chain polyunsaturated fatty acids, such as *arachidonic acid* and *eicosapentaenoic acid*, that play critical roles in immunity and inflammation.

Electrocardiogram (ECG or EKG). A recording of the electrical activity of the heart.

Electrolytes. Ionized salts in the body fluids, including sodium, potassium, magnesium, calcium and chloride.

Electron. A stable atomic particle with a negative charge.

Element. A chemical substance that can't be divided into simpler substances by chemical means.

Embolus. A blood clot.

Emergency Room (ER). The emergency department of a hospital.

Enamel. The hard, white, outermost layer of a tooth.

Endocrine system. The glands that secrete hormones, such as the *pituitary, thyroid, parathyroids, adrenals, pancreas, ovaries* and *testes.*

Endogenous. Arising from within the body.

Enzyme. A biological catalyst.

Epidemiological study. A study examining disease occurrence in a human population.

Epigenetics. The study of things that change how a gene behaves and may change the appearance or behaviour of cells but don't change the makeup of the gene itself.

Epigenome. That which controls the differential expression of genes in specific cells.

Epilepsy. A neurologic disorder characterized by repeated *seizures.*

Etiology. The cause of a disease.

Excretion. The elimination of wastes from blood or tissues.

Exercise. Light exercises are activities that do not cause breathlessness and burn 50 to 200 calories per hour. **Moderate exercises** use 200 to 350 calories per hour (ie. a brisk walk that leaves you slightly breathless but able to converse comfortably). **Vigorous exercises** require an exertion of over 350 calories per hour (ie. running, dancing the jive).

Fatty acid. An organic acid molecule consisting of a chain of carbon molecules and a carboxylic acid group found in fats, oils, phospholipids and *triglycerides.*

Fibrinogen. A critical agent in blood clotting.

Fixed eye deviation. The fixed gaze to right or left indicating the presence of brain trauma.

flavonoids. Powerful antioxidants that neutralize free radicals and prevent cellular damage that can lead to chronic diseases like cancer, heart disease, stroke and high blood pressure.

Free radical. A very reactive atom or molecule typically possessing a single unpaired electron.

Gene. A region of DNA that controls a specific hereditary characteristic.

Gene expression. The process by which the information coded in genes is converted to proteins and other cellular structures.

Genome. DNA.

Gingivitis. A non-destructive inflammation of the gums.

Glucose. A six-carbon sugar that is the major generator of energy for living organisms.

Glucose tolerance. The ability of the body to maintain normal glucose levels when challenged with a carbohydrate load.

Glutamate. An amino acid and the most common excitatory neurotransmitter in the brain.

Glycemic index (GI). An index of the blood glucose-raising potential of carbohydrates in a food.

Glycemic load (GL). An index that simultaneously describes the blood glucose-raising potential of the carbohydrates in a food and the quantity of carbohydrate in a food.

Glycogen. A large polymer of glucose molecules used to store energy in cells, especially muscle.

Glycoside. A compound containing a sugar molecule that can be broken by *hydrolysis* into a sugar and a nonsugar component (*aglycone*).

HDL (high density lipoproteins). A combination of fats and protein that transports cholesterol from tissues to the liver for elimination.

Hemiplegia. Paralysis of one side of the body.

Hemorrhage. Excessive or uncontrolled bleeding.

Hemorrhagic stroke. A stroke characterized by bleeding into the brain.

Homocysteine. A sulfur-containing amino acid.

Hormone. A chemical secreted by a gland which regulates the activity of specific cells.

Hydrolysis. Splitting a chemical bond in reaction to water.

Hypercholesterolemia. A high level of cholesterol in the blood, which is a precursor to many forms of disease, particularly those of the heart.

Hyperdense middle cerebral artery sign. A white area of increased density in M1 of the middle cerebral artery on a non-contrast CT scan of the head. It is one of the earliest and most useful signs of an intra-arterial blood clot causing ischemic stroke.

Hyperlipidemia. An excess quantity of fat (ie. *triglycerides, cholesterol*) in the bloodstream.

Hypertension (high blood pressure). Systolic blood pressure of 140 mm Hg or higher and/or a diastolic blood pressure of 90 mm Hg or higher.

Hypoglycemia. Low blood sugar, which may result in symptoms of sweating, trembling, hunger, dizziness, moodiness, confusion and blurred vision.

Hypothalamus. An area at the base of the brain that regulates bodily functions, such as body temperature, hunger and thirst.

Hypothesis. An educated guess proposed for further investigation.

Idiopathic. Of unknown cause.

Immunomodulator. A natural or synthetic substance that helps regulate or normalize the immune system.

Impaired glucose tolerance. A metabolic state between normal glucose regulation and overt diabetes.

Induction. Initiation of or increase in the expression of a gene in response to a physical or chemical stimulus.

Inflammation. A response to injury or infection.

Insulin. A hormone secreted by the beta-cells of the pancreas required for normal glucose metabolism.

Insulin resistance. Diminished responsiveness to insulin.

International normalized ratio (INR). The preferred method for reporting *prothrombin time*, which is a measure of blood coagulability.

Intervention trial. An experimental study used to test the effect of a treatment or intervention on a health- or disease-related outcome.

Intracellular fluid (ICF). The volume of fluid inside cells.

Intracranial hemorrhage. Bleeding within the skull.

Intermittent claudication. A condition characterized by leg pain or weakness on walkiing that diminishes or resolves with rest. It is usually associated with peripheral arterial disease.

In vitro. Research done in a test tube.

In vivo. Research done in a living organism.

Ion. A positive or negative electrically charged atomic particle.

Ischemia. A state of insufficient blood flow to a tissue.

Ischemic stroke. A stroke resulting from insufficient blood flow to an area of the brain.

IV (intravenous) bolus. A relatively large dose of medication administered into a vein over a short period of time.

Labetalol. A beta-blocker that also inhibits *alpha-adrenergic receptors (α-adrenergic receptors)* and safely lowers blood pressure rapidly, usually within about five minutes.

Lacunar stroke. A small ischemic stroke caused by the blockage of a small blood vessel in the brain; the most common effect is weakness or disability on one side of the body.

LDL (low density lipoprotein). A combination of fats and proteins that transports cholesterol from the liver to the tissues of the body.

Lipase. An enzyme secreted in the digestive tract that motivates the breakdown of large fat molecules (*triglycerides*) into individual fatty acids that can then be absorbed into the bloodstream.

Lipids. A chemical term for fats, including fatty acids, phospholipids, triglycerides and cholesterol.

Lipoproteins. Particles composed of fats and protein that carry cholesterol through the bloodstream.

Lumbar puncture. A spinal "tap" in which spinal fluid is collected through a needle from the subarachnoid space of the spinal cord for diagnostic or therapeutic purposes.

Magnetic Resonance Imaging (MRI). An imaging technique that uses a magnet and a computer to produce a picture of soft tissues.

Malignant. Cancerous.

Melatonin. A natural hormone secreted mostly by the pineal gland located in the centre of the brain and is not only a powerful hypnotic but is also a strong antioxidant, antidepressant, and *immunomodulator*.

Meta-analysis. A statistical technique combining results from several studies to obtain a quantitative estimate of the overall effect of a particular intervention or treatment.

Metabolism. The process by which a substance is assimilated and incorporated into the body.

Metabolite. A product from the metabolism of a compound.

Methionine. A sulfur-containing amino acid.

Micronutrient. A nutrient required by the body in small amounts, such as a vitamin or a mineral.

Migraine. A type of headache probably related to the abnormal sensitivity of arteries in the brain to various triggers, resulting in spasm and dilatation of the blood vessels.

mg/dl. Milligrams per decilitre.

mm Hg (millimeters of mercury). Unit of measure for blood pressure.

Monounsaturated fatty acid. A fatty acid with only one double bond between carbon atoms.

Multifactorial. Caused by several factors.

Multi-infarct dementia. Dementia associated with multiple strokes.

Mutation. A change in a gene.

Myelin. The fatty covering of nerve fibres.

Myelin-associated glycoprotein (MAG). A protein specific to the brain that prevents the growth of new nerve fibres needed to connect nerve cells. Levels of this protein are reduced by exercising regularly.

Myocardial infarction. A heart attack.

Myocardium. The heart muscle.

Myoglobin. An iron containing pigment in muscles.

Myopathy. Any disease of the muscles.

N-acylphosphatidylethanolamine (NAPE). A chemical messenger secreted by the small intestine after a meal that signals the satiety centre in your brain to stop eating.

National Institute of Health Stroke Scale (NIHSS) score. A 15-item neurological examination scale for stroke, used to measure several aspects of brain function, including consciousness, speech, vision, eye movement, motor strength, coordination and sensation. An experienced examiner should be able to rate the NIHSS of a stroke patient in 10 minutes or less. Ratings for each item are scored with three to five grades, with zero as normal. A maximum score of 42 represents a massive stroke from which the victim rarely recovers. An NIHSS of four or less indicates a minor stroke and suggests that tPA is not needed, whereas an NIHSS score equal to or greater than 21 signifies a severe stroke with the attendant excessive risk of serious bleeding complications from tPA treatment.

Necrosis. Cell death.

Need to treat (NNT). The number of patients who need to be treated in order to prevent one additional bad outcome (i.e. the number of patients that need to be treated for one to benefit compared with a control in a clinical trial).

Neurodegenerative. The degeneration or deterioration of nerve cells.

Neurologic. Involving nerves or the nervous system.

Neuron. A nerve cell that conducts nerve impulses, processing and transmitting information.

Neuropathy. Nerve damage or disease.

Neuroplasticity (or Cortical remapping). The ability of the human brain to change based on experience.

Neurotoxic. Damaging to nervous tissue.

Neurotransmitter. A chemical released from a nerve cell, usually resulting in the transmission of an impulse to another cell.

NIH. National Institutes of Health (of the United States of America).

Nitric oxide. A gas that promotes widening of the arteries.

Nogo-A. A protein specific to the brain that prevents the growth of new nerve fibres needed to connect nerve cells. Levels of this protein are reduced by exercising regularly.

Nucleic acid. Long polymers of nucleotides.

Nucleotides. Subunits of nucleic acids.

Nucleus. A membrane-bound cellular organelle containing DNA organized into chromosomes.

Nutrient. A chemical needed by an organism to live and grow or a substance taken in from the organism's environment and used for metabolism. Nutrients build and repair tissues, regulate body processes and are converted to and used as energy.

Nutrigenomics. The study of how the interaction between genetics and nutrition affects human health.

Obesity. More than average fatness. Having a *Body Mass Index (BMI)* greater than 30.

Observational study. A research in which participants are observed over time.

Obtundation. Less than full mental capacity in a medical patient, typically as a result of a medical condition or trauma. Also, a decreased level of alertness or consciouness.

Omega-3 fatty acids. Special fat components benefitting many functions of the human body.

Optimum health. Freedom from disease, plus maximum physical and mental fitness.

Organic. Of or relating to an organism, a living entity. Carbon-containing compounds. Agriculture using only natural fertilizers and non-chemical means of pest control.

Oxidant. A chemical agent that oxidizes.

Oxidation. A chemical reaction that removes electrons from an atom or molecule.

Oxidative stress. A condition in which pro-oxidants (e.g. free radicals) overwhelm antioxidants.

ParticipACTION. A national non-profit Canadian organization that promotes healthy living and physical fitness.

Patent foramen ovale. A congenital defect that allows blood clots in the right half of the heart, which should normally go to the lungs, to detour to the left side of the heart and from there to the brain, causing stroke.

Pathogen. A disease-causing agent, such as a bacteria.

Pathophysiology. The study of abnormal body functions or functions altered by disease.

Peptic ulcer. A disease characterized by ulcers in the inner lining of the stomach or *duodenum*.

Pericarditis. An inflammation of the pericardium or sac surrounding the heart.

Periodontitis. A destructive inflammation of the gums due to *plaque*, a film of bacteria and food particles deposited on the surfaces of teeth.

Peripheral arterial disease. *Atherosclerosis* of the arteries of the arms and legs.

Peripheral neuropathy. A disease or degenerative state affecting the nerves of the arms and legs.

Peripheral vascular disease. *Atherosclerosis* of the vessels of the arms and legs.

pH. A measure of acidity or alkalinity.

Pharmacokinetics. The study of the absorption, distribution, metabolism and elimination of drugs.

Pharmaconogsy. The study of medicines derived from natural sources.

Pharmacologic dose. The amount of a nutrient or drug enough for the maintenance of health.

Phase I clinical trial. An experiment to determine the bioavailability, optimal dose and safety of a new therapy.

Phase II clinical trial. An experiment to investigate the effectiveness and safety of a new therapy.

Phlebotomy. The removal of blood from a vein.

Photosynthesis. The process that plants with chorophyll use to transform carbon dioxide, water and light into organic compounds, particularly carbohydrates and oxygen.

Physical fitness. A state of healthy well-being that allows an individual to live a good quality of life.

Phytochemicals. Biologically active compounds synthesized by plants.

Phytoestrogens. Compounds with estrogenic activity derived from plants.

Pigment. A compound that gives a plant or animal cell colour.

Pituitary gland. An *endocrine gland* at the base of the brain.

Placebo. An inert treatment given to a control group while the experimental group is given the active treatment.

Placebo-controlled study. A research conducted to make sure that the result is due to the experimental treatment.

Plasma. The liquid portion of blood.

Plasminogin. A substance naturally produced by the body that helps break down blood clots.

Platelet. Cell fragments that assist in blood clotting.

Platelet anti-aggregant. A medication or other substance that prevents blood clotting.

Polymorphism. A variant form of a gene.

Polyunsaturated fatty acid. A fatty acid with more than one double bond between carbons.

Positron Emission Tomography (PET) scan. A diagnostic imaging technique that shows the difference between healthy and abnormally functioning tissues.

Potassium. A dietary mineral critical to the human body.

Precursor. The predecessor of a particular product.

Prehypertension. Blood pressure elevated above normal but not to the level considered to be *hypertension* (high blood pressure). A *systolic pressure* of 120 to 139 and/or a *diastolic pressure* of 80 to 89.

Prognosis. The predicted outcome based on the course of a disease.

Pro-oxidant. An atom or molecule that promotes the oxidation of another atom or molecule by accepting electrons.

Prophylaxis. The treatment used to prevent a disease.

Prospective cohort study. An observational research in which a group of people (a cohort) is interviewed or tested for risk factors and then followed up at subsequent times to determine their health status.

Prostaglandins. Cell-signaling molecules involved in inflammation.

Protein. A complex organic molecule composed of amino acids in a specific order.

Proton. A positively charged elementary particle.

Randomized controlled trial (RCT). A clinical research in which participants are unknowingly and indiscriminately selected to receive either the active treatment or a placebo.

Receptor. A specialized molecule of a cell that binds a specific chemical.

Recessive trait. A trait that is expressed only when two copies of the gene responsible for the trait are present.

Restenosis. The renarrowing of an artery after it has been dilated.

Retina. The nerve layer in the back of the eye where images created by light are converted to nerve impulses and transmitted via the optic nerve to the brain.

Retrospective study. An *epidemiological study* that begins after the exposure and the disease have occurred.

Ruminant. An animal that chews cud, such as cattle, sheep and deer.

Salicylates. Compounds of salicylic acid derived from the bark of willow tree, the natural source of aspirin.

Saturated fatty acid. A fatty acid with no double bonds between carbon atoms.

Seizure. Uncontrolled electrical activity in the brain, usually leading to a convulsion.

Serum. The liquid portion of blood, minus clotting factors.

Silent stroke. Small strokes that do not cause any symptoms but that can still damage brain tissue.

Statin myopathy. An inflammation of the muscles caused by a statin medication. The most severe form causes destruction of the muscle tissue, called *rhabdomyolysis*. The most common symptoms of statin myopathy include muscle pain and muscle weakness. Additional symptoms of worsening statin myopathy include muscle swelling, and pink, red or brown urine. Treatment for severe *rhabdomyolysis* may include kidney dialysis.

Stenosis. The obstruction or narrowing of a passage, usually of an artery.

Steroid. A molecule related to cholesterol.

Stroke. Damage that occurs to a part of the brain when its blood supply is suddenly interrupted.

Stroke risk factors. High blood pressure. Smoking. Abdominal obesity. Unhealthy diet. Physical inactivity. High cholesterol. Diabetes. Alcohol abuse. Stress/depression. Heart disease.

Subarachnoid hemorrhage. A rare type of stroke caused by bleeding into the space under the arachnoid membrane of the brain, most commonly from trauma or from the rupture of an aneurysm.

Subclinical. The time before clinical signs or symptoms are detectable by clinical examination or laboratory tests.

Substrate. A reactant in an enzyme-catalyzed reaction.

Supplement. A nutrient provided in addition to that which is available in the diet.

Syndrome. A combination of symptoms indicative of a specific disease.

Synergistic. The benefit of two treatments together being greater than the sum of the effects of the two individual treatments.

Synthesis. The formation of a chemical compound from its precursors.

Systematic review. A structured review of the literature designed to answer a specific question.

Systolic blood pressure. The upper number in a blood pressure reading, which represents the highest arterial pressure measured during the heartbeat cycle.

Tai chi chuan. The ancient Chinese system of gentle movement patterns.

Thermic effect. The calories expended by our bodies to eat and digest the foods we consume.

Thrombolytic. A clot-busting drug.

Thrombotic stroke. Caused by blood clots.

Tissue Plasmogen Activator (tPA). A drug used in the treatment of acute stroke.

Tocopherols (TCP). A series of organic chemical compounds of which many have Vitamin E activity. Also, *a-tocopherol* or *alpha-tocopherol*.

Tocotrienols. Compounds related to *tocopherols* which also have vitamin E activity. All of these various derivatives with vitamin activity may correctly be referred to as "Vitamin E." *Tocopherols* and *tocotrienols* are fat-soluble antioxidants but also seem to have other functions in the body as well.

Transient ischemic attack (TIA). A warning or mini stroke.

Transient global anemia. Temporary but almost total disruption of the memory.

Triglycerides. Lipids consisting of three fatty acid molecules bound to a *glycerol*.

Ultrasonography. A test using high-frequency sound waves to produce a picture.

Unsaturated fatty acid. A fatty acid with at least one double bond between carbons.

Vascular dementia. Dementia resulting from *cerebrovascular disease*.

Vascular endothelium. The single cell layer that lines the inner surface of blood vessels.

Vasoconstriction. The narrowing of a blood vessel.

Vasodilation. The relaxation or opening of a blood vessel.

Ventricles. The two lower chambers of the heart that pump blood to the body (left) and the lungs (right).

Vitamin. An organic compound necessary for normal physiological function.

Warfarin. An anticoagulant drug.

Whispering stroke. Strokes with symptoms that are so mild that they are easily ignored.

A

B

C

H

I

L

M

N

additional reading

Ultimate Fitness: The Quest for Truth about Health and Exercise.
Gina Kolata. Farrar Straus and Giroux. 2003.

In Defense of Food: An Eater's Manifesto.
Michael Pollan. Penguin Press. 2008.

Meditation As Medicine: Activate the Power of Your Natural Healing Force.
Dharma Singh Khalsa and Cameron Stauth. Atria. 2002.

Easy Way To Stop Smoking: New Canadian Edition.
Allen Carr. Clarity Pubishing. 2004.

Overdosed America: The Broken Promised of American Medicine.
John Abramson, M. D. HarperCollins Publishers. 2004.

The DASH Diet Action Plan.
Marla Heller, M.S., R. D. Amidon Press. 2007.

Happy At Last (The Thinking Person's Guide to Finding Joy).
Dr.Richard O'Connor, M.S.W., Ph.D. St. Martin's Press. 2008.